Jennifer H. Peterson, DVM (signature)

Neurological Examination for the Busy Practitioner

Mary O. Smith

BVM&S, PhD, MRCVS, Diplomate ACVIM (Neuro~

Illustrations by Michelle M.

Library of Congress Cataloging-in-Publication Data

on file

ISBN 1-58326-034-X

Contents

List of Tables

List of Figures

Introduction

The life of the practicing veterinarian is a busy and demanding one. Finding time to perform a thorough examination of a patient with neurological signs when one has several other patients in the waiting room can seem a daunting task. Performing a complete neurological examination is not an opportunity the general practitioner has every day, so it is easy to feel one's skills may be "rusty." Yet, the exam can take little more than ten minutes, and a few guidelines can help restore the examiner's confidence. The neurological examination is the most important step in clinical neurology, because it is the key to neuroanatomic localization of lesions and thereby to differential diagnosis and a diagnostic plan.

The inspiration for this guide comes from the many practitioners I talk with on a daily basis. What they often need is a little guidance and a reminder of the principles and practice of neurological examination. How do you manage when your patient is a 160-pound St. Bernard or a frightened and uncooperative Siamese cat? Exactly where do you need to percuss the limb to test the triceps reflex, and what does that reflex tell you? I hope that this guide will help practitioners and thereby help their clients and, most importantly, their patients.

This book is intended to be a practical guide to performing and interpreting a neurological examination of cats and dogs. It is not an exhaustive text, nor a replacement for the several excellent textbooks on the clinical neurology of small animals; this book is intended to be used as a complementary reference for the practicing clinician. There is no mention, therefore, of differential diagnosis, specific diagnosis, or treatment of neurological disease. The information in this book is presented using a step-by-step approach, which I hope will be helpful to veterinarians who do not perform neurological examinations every day. The included details of neuroanatomy are brief, covering only those points essential for the reader to understand how the results of examination facilitate neuroanatomic localization of lesions. Several textbooks of small animal neurology and neuroanatomy are listed in Appendix 3.

The techniques described in this guide are based on my sixteen years of experience as a veterinary clinical neurologist, and I make no claims for them being "better" than those suggested by other authors. They have proven reliable for me, however, and I hope they will help my readers.

When information in this text refers both to males and females, animal patients are referred to as male. This does not imply any gender prejudice, but simply avoids the cumbersome necessity of always referring to both sexes.

I am indebted to Dr. Michelle Murray for her excellent illustrations that serve to further clarify the text.

The Purpose of the Neurological Examination

There is a tendency to think of the nervous system as the most "hidden" of all organ systems, because it cannot be easily visualized or biopsied. It can be argued, however, that the nervous system is the most visible of all organ systems, because its function is revealed in every action taken by an animal and in every response to external stimuli.

The neurological examination answers the following two questions:

- Is neurological disease present?

- Where is the disease process located within the nervous system?

Most animals with neurological disease have abnormalities that can be observed during the neurological examination. Occasionally, the neurological examination may be normal, even when neurological disease is present; an example is an animal with seizures. In such a case, historical information may be the main indicator that the patient has neurological disease. It is often possible to determine the severity of the neurological dysfunction to some extent by subjectively quantitating the severity of neurological dysfunction. An animal with hind-limb paralysis, for example, has more severe disease than an animal with paresis of the hind limbs. Prognosis similarly may be estimated by quantitating the severity of the abnormality. One should be cautious, however, in extrapolating information about disease severity and prognosis from the results of a single neurological examination, which is merely a "snapshot" of nervous system function. Examinations repeated over time are more helpful in the assessment of disease progression and prognosis.

WHEN TO PERFORM A NEUROLOGICAL EXAMINATION

Clinicians perform a large part of the neurological examination every time they carry out a complete physical examination. Mental status, posture, gait, cranial nerve (CN) function, and muscle mass and tone are routinely assessed as part of the physical examination. Abnormal findings in any one of these areas signify the need for a detailed determination of neurological function. Historical information, such as a history of seizures or exercise intolerance, may also suggest that neurological disease is present and may prompt more detailed investigation. A neurological examination takes but a few minutes. With practice and experience, this examination can reveal more about the functional status of the nervous system than the most advanced diagnostic techniques. Therefore, the guiding principle should be, "If neurological disease crosses your mind, do a neurological examination."

LIMITATIONS OF THE NEUROLOGICAL EXAMINATION

Interpretation of the findings of neurological examination is somewhat subjective. Subtle deficits, such as mild sensory loss or slight changes in mentation, may be impossible to detect. Furthermore, the accuracy of the findings depends in part on the experience level of the examiner. There is a considerable range of normal neurological function, varying with factors such as the age, species, breed, and anxiety level of the animal. The greater the experience of the examiner, the more capable he or she is of interpreting the neurological examination results as being within or outside the normal range. Practice makes better, if not perfect, especially when it comes to the neurological examination.

Always carry out a complete neurological examination, so that the functioning of the nervous system can be interpreted in its entirety. A single clinical finding may be interpreted in different ways when viewed in relation to other findings. Animals with lateralized vestibular disease and those with lateralized cerebral disease, for example, may exhibit similar tendencies to circle in one direction. The findings on the remainder of the neurological examination enable the veterinarian to differentiate between the two. The various components of the neurological examination can be thought of as different colors in a painting; one needs to be able to see all the colors to recognize the subject of the picture.

CONDITIONS FOR NEUROLOGICAL EXAMINATION

Animals' responses are altered by factors such as fear and anxiety. It is best to carry out a neurological examination in a quiet, calm, and nonthreatening environment. Sedatives, anesthetics, and other neuro-active drugs profoundly change nervous system function and should not be used in animals that are to undergo a neurological examination. When an animal has already received such medications, the results of the neurological examination should be interpreted with great caution, and the examination should be repeated once the effects of the drugs have worn off.

2

Preliminaries to the Neurological Examination

CHIEF COMPLAINT

The chief complaint often suggests the location of the neurological lesion, or it may be consistent with disease in several areas of the nervous system. Seizures indicate brain involvement. Generalized weakness, however, can be the result of a lesion in the brain, the spinal cord, the peripheral nerves, or the muscles. Table 1 lists common signs of neurological disease and the likely locations of lesions causing those signs. Table 2 lists the signs that typically result from lesions at various locations within the nervous system.

SIGNALMENT

Many neurological diseases are more prevalent in animals of a certain species, breed, or age. Canine distemper virus infection, for example, occurs in dogs but not in cats. Acute intervertebral disk protrusion is common in dachshunds and other chondrodystrophoid dog breeds, but it is unusual in terriers and hounds. Other diseases occur more

TABLE 1

Common Signs of Neurological Disease and Corresponding Locations of Lesions Within the Nervous System

Clinical Sign	Nervous System Location
Dull mentation	Cerebrum; ARAS[1] in thalamus, midbrain, or medulla
Stupor or coma	Cerebrum; ARAS in thalamus, midbrain, or rostral medulla; coma more commonly due to ARAS lesion
Aggression, hysteria	Cerebrum or thalamus, involving limbic system
Seizures	Cerebrum; causes of seizures may be intracranial or extracranial
Blindness	Retina, optic nerve, optic chiasm, optic tract— primary ocular lesion; midbrain (lateral geniculate nucleus); cerebrum (occipital cortex), optic radiation
Mydriasis	Retina, optic nerve—primary ocular lesion; oculomotor nerve or nucleus (midbrain)
Miosis	Sympathetic nerve to the eye—primary ocular lesion (Horner's syndrome); cortical, thalamic, or early midbrain lesion
Decreased pupillary light reflex	Retina, optic nerve, optic chiasma, optic tract, midbrain (lateral geniculate nucleus), oculomotor nerve—primary ocular lesion
Circling	Cerebrum or thalamus; midbrain; vestibular system (central or peripheral)
Opisthotonus	Midbrain—decerebrate posture; cerebellum— decerebellate posture
Head turn	Cerebrum, thalamus—ipsiversive head turn
Head tilt	Vestibular system (central or peripheral)
Leaning or falling to one side	Vestibular system (central or peripheral)
Nystagmus	Vestibular system (central or peripheral)

TABLE 1 (continued)

Common Signs of Neurological Disease and Corresponding Locations of Lesions Within the Nervous System

Clinical Sign	Nervous System Location
Strabismus	Cranial nerve III; constant and ventrolateral Cranial nerve VI; constant and medial Vestibular system; changes in direction or in body position
Quadriparesis	Brain stem or spinal cord C_1-C_5; with increased reflexes in all four limbs Spinal cord C_6-T_2; with decreased forelimb and increased hind-limb reflexes Diffuse or multifocal spinal cord; multiple peripheral nerves; muscle; neuromuscular junction; with decreased reflexes in all four limbs
Hemiparesis	Contralateral cerebrum or midbrain; ipsilateral brain stem or spinal cord C_1-C_5; with increased reflexes in both limbs on affected side Ipsilateral spinal cord C_6-T_2; with decreased forelimb and increased hind limb reflexes on affected side
Paraparesis	Spinal cord T_3-L_3; with increased reflexes in both hind limbs Spinal cord L_4-S_2 or peripheral nerves; with decreased reflexes on both hind limbs
Paresis or lameness in one limb	Local spinal cord segments; peripheral nerve; muscle
Muscle atrophy	Peripheral nerves; muscle; neuromuscular junction (uncommon)
Tremors	Cerebellum—intention tremor Numerous possible sites in either central or peripheral nervous system—other tremors
Decreased or absent pain perception	Spinal cord (any level), peripheral nerve; loss of sensation is distal to the lesion
Urinary incontinence	Spinal cord rostral to S_1, brain; bladder with good tone and difficult to express Spinal cord S_1-S_3, peripheral nerve; flaccid bladder, easy to express
Fecal incontinence	Spinal cord S_1-S_3, peripheral nerves

[1] ARAS = Ascending Reticular Activating System

TABLE 2

**Summary of Clinical Signs Resulting From Lesions
at Various Sites in the Nervous System**

Lesion Location	Clinical Signs
Cerebrum and thalamus	Changes in behavior and mentation; seizures; normal gait on a level surface with ataxia and paresis on slopes, stairs; contralateral proprioceptive and postural reaction deficits; myotactic reflexes normal to increased in contralateral limbs; ipsiversive circling; ipsiversive head turn (occasional); small pupils, responsive to light (occasional)
Limbic system (cerebral, thalamic, hypothalamic, and midbrain centers)	Changes in behavior—increased or decreased aggression, altered sexual behavior, changes in appetite and thirst, seizures (often bizarre)
Midbrain	Moderate to severely decreased mentation; decerebrate posture; mild/early lesions—small pupils; severe lesions—dilated pupils with loss of pupillary light reflex and oculocephalic reflex; compulsive circling; contralateral hemiparesis to paralysis, ataxia, proprioceptive and postural reaction deficits; myotactic reflexes normal to increased in contralateral limbs; head tilt away from lesion (rare)
Medulla oblongata	Deficits in any of the cranial nerves V-XII; head tilt and spontaneous nystagmus; decreased mentation (occasional); ipsilateral hemiparesis to paralysis, ataxia; proprioceptive and postural reaction deficits; myotactic reflexes normal to increased in ipsilateral limbs
Cerebellum	Intention tremor; ataxia in ipsilateral limbs; hypermetria; decreased to absent menace reflex; increased myotactic reflexes in ipsilateral limbs
Cranial nerves (peripheral)	A wide range of signs of dysfunction on the ipsilateral side of the head

TABLE 2 (continued)

Summary of Clinical Signs Resulting From Lesions at Various Sites in the Nervous System

Lesion Location	Clinical Signs
Spinal cord C_1-C_5	Ipsilateral ataxia and paresis to paralysis in fore- and hind limbs, with normal to increased reflexes; possible urinary incontinence with upper-motor neuron-type bladder dysfunction
Spinal cord C_6-T_2	Ipsilateral ataxia and paresis to paralysis in fore- and hind limbs with decreased reflexes in the forelimbs and normal to increased reflexes in the hind limbs; +/- ipsilateral Horner's syndrome (preganglionic); +/- ipsilateral loss of the panniculus reflex; +/- urinary incontinence with upper-motor neuron-type bladder dysfunction
Spinal cord T_3-L_3	Ipsilateral ataxia and paresis to paralysis in hind limbs with normal to increased reflexes; possible urinary incontinence with upper-motor neuron-type bladder dysfunction
Spinal cord L_4-S_2	Ipsilateral ataxia and paresis to paralysis in hind limbs with decreased reflexes; +/- urinary incontinence with lower-motor neuron-type bladder dysfunction
Spinal cord S_1-S_3; cauda equina	Flaccid paresis to paralysis of the tail; urinary incontinence with lower-motor neuron-type bladder dysfunction; flaccid paresis to paralysis of the anus, with fecal incontinence
Peripheral somatic nerves	Paresis to paralysis of one limb (focal lesions), or several limbs (diffuse disease); rapid muscle atrophy; loss of sensation in limbs; paresthesia (occasional)
Neuromuscular junction; muscles	Weakness; exercise intolerance; muscle atrophy (less common)

commonly in animals within a specific age group; for example, feline infectious peritonitis occurs more often in young cats, and central nervous system (CNS) neoplasia is seen in middle-aged to older cats. While it is essential not to approach any patient with a rigidly preconceived idea of the eventual diagnosis, knowing the likely prevalence of specific diseases in animals with a particular signalment is helpful when making a list of differential diagnoses and planning the diagnostic workup.

HISTORY

Just as certain diseases tend to affect specific types of animals, so, too, do they tend to follow certain clinical courses. Acute or peracute onset of disease with little progression, or even some resolution, suggests a traumatic or vascular etiology. A chronic, progressive course is seen with degenerative diseases, such as degenerative myelopathy of German shepherd dogs. Some disease processes, such as infectious diseases, can have either acute or gradual onset and variable progression of disease. Finally, acute events may be superimposed on chronic, progressive disease, such as a hemorrhage within or adjacent to a neoplasm. In this last case, the signs of the chronic disease may be subtle or inapparent, and the animal is presented for signs that are recent and acute in onset. As with information concerning signalment, historical data can be used to help develop a list of differential diagnoses upon which the choice of subsequent diagnostic tests can be based.

Historical information may be important in linking other manifestations of disease to the neurological problem. A dog presented for recent onset of seizures may also have a history of polydipsia, polyuria, and weakness. All these clinical signs might be seen in a dog with a pituitary tumor producing both secondary hyperadrenocorticism and the seizure disorder. Coughing and dyspnea in an animal presented for altered mentation and behavior might suggest metastatic neoplasia as a possible cause for both the respiratory and CNS signs.

PHYSICAL EXAMINATION

Neurological examination should always be preceded by a thorough physical examination. Many diseases that affect the nervous system are organ specific and rarely cause systemic disease. Systemic diseases, however, may secondarily affect the nervous system. A dog presented for the complaint of neck pain may be found to have mucosal petechiation and a fever—both suggestive of *Ehrlichia canis* infection, which can also cause meningitis. Conjunctivitis in a young puppy with seizures may suggest canine distemper infection. Several diseases that affect the CNS may also affect the eyes, so a complete ophthalmological examination should be a part of any neurological examination. Occasionally, animals with signs that appear to be of nervous system origin may have non-neurological disease. Such is the case in dogs with bilateral cranial cruciate ligament rupture and cats with "saddle" thrombus, which are often presented with a complaint of acute-onset "paraplegia." It is important not to jump to conclusions when examining an animal with neurological disease, and a thorough physical examination may reveal vital information.

Neurological examination should be carried out in a consistent manner. However, each veterinarian should develop his or her own preferred technique. A summary of neurological examination procedures is given in Appendix 1.

3

Assessment of Mental Status and Behavior

The neurological examination should always begin with an assessment of the patient's mental status (i.e., mentation) and behavior. This is easily done before the physical examination, while taking a history. The patient should be allowed to wander freely around the room while his reactions to the unfamiliar surroundings are observed.

NORMAL FINDINGS

Appropriate reactions range from curiosity and active exploration of the room to anxiety and a desire to stay close to the owner. Some behaviors are appropriate for certain breeds but not others. Breeds of dog known to be outgoing and gregarious tend to be more adventurous, while cats and small or toy breeds of dog may be more anxious. Puppies and kittens behave differently from adult dogs and cats. Behavior also depends on individual personality as well as previous experience, such as whether the animal is often taken outside the home. Even aggressive behavior, although not desirable, may be considered normal in some circumstances.

ABNORMAL FINDINGS

Abnormal mental status includes all of the following: undue fear, anxiety, or aggression; dullness or depression; excessive sleepiness; and blunted or absent responses to external stimuli such as movement, noise, and physical handling. Animals with decreased mental awareness can be classified as follows:

- Dull, lethargic, or obtunded. The animal's interest in his surroundings is mildly to moderately reduced. His responses to visual, auditory, and tactile stimuli are decreased, and he may appear to be sleepy. These descriptive terms encompass a wide range of severity of clinical signs. Depression often denotes a similar mental state, but more properly refers to a psychological condition in humans, which does not occur in animals.

- Stupor. The animal appears to be asleep, but he can be roused by vigorous stimuli, such as a pinch, a loud noise, or handling.

- Coma. The animal appears to be asleep and cannot be roused even by painful stimuli. Reflex responses such as withdrawal of the limb in response to a pinch of the toe may be present in comatose animals, but the patient does not become alert in response to such stimuli. "Unconscious" is another descriptive term for animals that are comatose. Comatose patients also may have abnormal posture, specifically, decerebrate rigidity (see below).

CLINICAL NEUROANATOMY

Mental awareness is the function of the higher centers of the brain, particularly the cerebral cortex and the ascending reticular activating system (ARAS).

The cerebral cortex is the most recently developed, and phylogenetically it is the youngest part of the CNS. It is much better developed in mammals than in other animals, and it reaches its peak of development in primates. Sensory information reaches the level of consciousness in the cerebral cortex, and voluntary movements are initiated there.

The ARAS consists of groups of nerve cell bodies and axons located centrally—like the core of an apple—throughout the rostral medulla oblongata, the midbrain, and the thalamus. Sensory information from the body and head is carried by the ARAS and diffusely projected to the cerebral cortex, where it reaches the level of consciousness. Not all sensory input to the cerebrum travels in the ARAS, but ARAS activity is essential for maintaining consciousness. Both cerebral and ARAS lesions cause similar clinical signs, and it may be difficult to distinguish absolutely between the two on the basis of neurological examination findings. A general rule of thumb is that lesions of the ARAS tend to cause more severe clinical abnormalities than lesions in the cerebrum.

Lateralized cerebral or ARAS lesions cause other unilateral or asymmetrical neurological signs in the head and body, in addition to decreased mental awareness. These include circling, decreased proprioceptive and postural reactions in the limbs opposite the side of the lesion, and blindness in the opposite visual field. Signs of cerebral and midbrain ARAS lesions are compared in Table 3.

Lesions in either the cerebrum or the midbrain also affect sensory functions. The animal has decreased awareness of a variety of stimuli on the side of the body opposite the lesion. This most often appears as decreased response to tactile stimulation of the face, which can be mistaken for a lesion of CN V. In more severe cases, animals ignore stimuli such as food presented on the side opposite the lesion. When food is presented to the side of the head ipsilateral to the lesion, the animal can locate it and will eat. When food is presented to the side of the head contralateral to the lesion, the animal may smell the food and seek it, but he does not turn toward the food and is unable to locate it. This situation of ignoring the side of the world contralateral to a cerebral or midbrain lesion is called hemi-inattention syndrome.

Altered behavior, such as increased aggression or affection, excessive fear, or changes in sexual behavior, may result from lesions in the limbic system. The limbic system is comprised of centers in the temporal lobe of the cerebrum and various groups of nerve cells (i.e., nuclei) in the thalamus, hypothalamus, and midbrain. The limbic system is involved in the control of emotion and very basic behaviors such as

TABLE 3

Comparison of Cerebral and Midbrain ARAS[1] Lesions

Neurological Signs	Cerebral Disease	Midbrain Disease
Consciousness	Mildly decreased consciousness to coma	Mildly decreased consciousness to coma; more likely to cause stupor and coma
Posture	No abnormal posture	Decerebrate rigidity; head tilt away from lesion (rare)
Vision	Contralateral blindness	Contralateral blindness
Pupil size and PLR[2]	Pupils normal to small; PLR present	Pupils small in early/mild lesions; dilated, nonresponsive pupils in severe lesions
Oculocephalic reflex	Present	Reduced to absent
Position of severe globes	Normal	Ventrolateral strabismus in disease
Circling	Toward side of lesion; mild to strong tendency	Toward side of lesion; compulsive
Gait on a level surface	Minimal to no deficits observed	Contralateral paresis and ataxia
Gait on a slope, stairs, etc.	Contralateral paresis and ataxia	Contralateral paresis and ataxia
Proprioception and postural reactions	Decreased to absent in contralateral limbs	Decreased to absent in contralateral limbs

[1] ARAS = Ascending Reticular Activating System
[2] PLR = Pupillary Light Reflex(es)

eating, drinking, aggression, and sexual function. Limbic system lesions may cause profound behavioral changes

CLINICAL TIPS

- Observe mental status before doing any part of the physical or neurological examination. This will permit the best assessment of the patient's "resting" level of consciousness.

- Some normal animals may be so fearful that they will hide under a chair. In such cases, try removing from the room objects that offer hiding places. Moving to a different site, such as an outside area, may help.

- Question the owner about whether the animal's behavior has changed in any way.

- Historical information about behavior may reveal abnormalities not detected in the examination room. It can be helpful to have owners record on video the abnormal behavior or mentation in the pet that occurs at home.

- Animals may have episodes of abnormal behavior, rather than continuous clinical signs. Underlying problems causing episodic abnormalities include intermittent toxicities (e.g., drug or toxic plant exposure), fluctuating metabolic disease (e.g., hepatic encephalopathy), or seizure-related phenomena. The abnormal behavior may itself be a form of seizure activity, or it may be postictal activity. When owners do not observe the onset of the abnormal episodes but find the animal already in the abnormal condition, postictal activity should be suspected. Seizures can occur unobserved, and then the owner finds the animal in a confused, dull, postictal state. Question the owner about other seizure-related events, such as urine or feces found in the house.

- Increased intracranial pressure, which has many etiologies, is a common underlying cause of cerebral and ARAS dysfunction.

4

Posture and Attitude

Observe the position of the head, limbs, and body in space. Posture and attitude can be evaluated throughout the neurological examination and while the animal is stationary, moving, and ascending and descending stairs.

NORMAL FINDINGS

- Normal animals stand with the head erect and body weight distributed approximately equally on all four limbs. The head faces forward, and the base of each ear is the same distance from the ground.

- In response to noise, movement, or other stimuli, the animal may turn his head or cock his head to one side, but he will not maintain these positions for long.

- When standing and facing up a slope or ascending stairs, the forelimbs will be relatively flexed and the hind limbs will be relatively extended. The reverse is true when the animal is facing down a slope or descending stairs.

- When standing at rest on a level surface, the animal's back should be level, with shoulders and hips approximately the same distance from the ground.

- The righting reaction is the natural tendency of an animal to rise from a position of lateral recumbency. This is checked later in the neurological examination, subsequent to examination of the myotactic reflexes.

- During testing of the reflexes, the animal is held in lateral recumbency, first on one side, then on the other. In each case, the animal should rise immediately when he is released, to a position where the back is dorsal and the head is upright.

ABNORMAL FINDINGS

Animals with neurological disease may adopt a variety of abnormal postures.

Head Tilt

- Head tilt is the most common abnormal posture seen in animals with neurological disease.

- A head tilt is present when one ear is held lower than the other. The tilt is described as being toward the side of the ear that is held closer to the ground.

- A head tilt is a rotation of the head around its sagittal axis; that is, from the front to the back of the head.

- Head tilt almost always indicates vestibular disease, and other signs of vestibular dysfunction usually accompany head tilt, such as circling and nystagmus (Table 4).

Head Turn

- A head turn exists when the head is held with the nose turned back toward the flank.

TABLE 4

Clinical Signs of Vestibular Disease

Clinical Signs	Location of Lesion Within the Vestibular System		
	Peripheral	Central	Paradoxical (Cerebellum)
Circling and falling	Toward the side of the lesion	Toward the side of the lesion	Away from the side of the lesion
Head tilt	Toward the lesion	Toward the lesion	Away from the lesion
Nystagmus	Horizontal or rotatory; fast phase away from the lesion	Horizontal or rotatory; fast phase away from the lesion; also vertical, diagonal, disconjugate, positional	Horizontal or rotatory; fast phase toward the lesion; also vertical, diagonal, disconjugate, positional
Proprioceptive and postural reaction deficits	None	Ipsilateral to the lesion	Ipsilateral to the lesion
Cranial nerve deficits	+/- Cranial nerve VII; Horner's syndrome; ipsilateral to the lesion	+/- Cranial nerves V, VII-XII; ipsilateral to the lesion	+/- Cranial nerves V, VII-XII; ipsilateral to the lesion

Opisthotonus and Extensor Rigidity

- Opisthotonus is a posture where the head and neck are held in extreme extension. Extensor rigidity describes postures where the limbs are held stiffly, with all the joints extended. Extensor rigidity usually involves all four limbs or the forelimbs alone.

CLINICAL NEUROANATOMY

Head Tilt

- Head tilt almost always indicates vestibular disease.

- The head tilt is toward the side of the lesion in all cases of peripheral vestibular disease and most cases of central vestibular disease.

- When lesions involve the vestibular pathways in the cerebellum, head tilt may be away from the side of the lesion (Table 4).

- Very rarely, disruption of visual pathways within the midbrain causes severe head tilt away from the side of the lesion. Other signs of midbrain disease are present.

Head Turn

- Head turn is seen in cerebral and thalamic disease.

- The head turn is toward the side of the lesion.

- Head turn due to cerebral or thalamic lesions is accompanied by other signs, which may include some or all of the following:
  — Altered mental status
  — Postural and proprioceptive deficits in the contralateral limbs
  — Reduced vision or blindness in the opposite visual field
  — Circling toward the side of the lesion

- Rarely, head turn may be seen due to other causes, such as neck pain. A complete examination should help differentiate this from cerebral disease.

Opisthotonus

- When opisthotonus occurs in conjunction with extensor rigidity of all four limbs and markedly decreased mentation, it signifies midbrain disease. This posture is called decerebrate rigidity (below). When opisthotonus occurs in conjunction with extensor rigidity of the forelimbs, together with intention tremor and other evidence of cerebellar disease, the posture is called decerebellate rigidity. Extensor rigidity of the forelimbs without opisthotonus occurs in Schiff-Sherrington syndrome, the result of lesions affecting the thoracolumbar spinal cord.

Decerebrate Rigidity

- In decerebrate rigidity, all four limbs are rigidly extended and opisthotonus is present.

- Marked proprioceptive and postural reaction deficits are present in the limbs. Myotactic reflexes are normal to increased.

- Lesions in the midbrain that affect the ARAS cause decerebrate rigidity.

- Animals in decerebrate rigidity have severe mental dullness, usually to the extent of coma.

- Other signs of midbrain disease are present, such as marked mydriasis, absent or decreased pupillary light reflexes, and reduced or absent oculocephalic reflexes (i.e., physiological nystagmus).

Decerebellate Rigidity

- Animals with severe cerebellar lesions have opisthotonus and extensor rigidity of the forelimbs. The hind limbs usually are flexed or may show alternating extension and flexion movements. In very rare cases of almost complete cerebellar destruction, the hind limbs as well as the forelimbs may be rigidly extended.

- Animals with pure cerebellar lesions have normal consciousness and have other signs of cerebellar disease, such as intention tremor.

- When lesions involve the cerebellum alone, proprioceptive and postural reactions are normal in the limbs, although myotactic reflexes may be mildly increased.

- Lesions affecting the cerebellum often involve the medulla oblongata also. In this case, other signs of medulla disease are present, including ipsilateral paresis, ataxia, and postural and proprioceptive reaction deficits.

Schiff-Sherrington Syndrome

- This abnormal posture is not unusual in dogs with severe thoracolumbar spinal cord disease, but it is very rare in other species.

- Dogs with Schiff-Sherrington syndrome have extensor rigidity of the forelimbs without opisthotonus.

- Proprioception and postural reactions are normal in the forelimbs of dogs with Schiff-Sherrington syndrome, but they are decreased to absent in the hind limbs.

- Lesions of the spinal cord in the thoracolumbar area cause Schiff-Sherrington syndrome by interrupting an ascending pathway from the lumbar intumescence to the cervical intumescence. The function of this ascending pathway is to inhibit alpha motor neurons to forelimb extensor muscles. When the pathway is damaged, forelimb extension is disinhibited.

- Although the forelimb movements are stiff because of the increased extensor tone, postural and proprioceptive reactions in the forelimbs are normal, because there is no lesion at the level of or rostral to the origin of the nerves of the brachial plexus.

- The ascending inhibitory pathway involved in this phenomenon lies centrally in the spinal cord, adjacent to the spinal cord ventral horn gray matter. Lesions involving this pathway, therefore, tend to be fairly severe.

Abnormal Righting Reactions

- Animals with vestibular disease may not rise from lateral recumbency when the side of the lesion is toward the ground. They may vigorously resist lying with the lesion side uppermost.

- Animals that lose the righting reaction because they have vestibular disease must be distinguished from those that are too weak to rise because of spinal cord or neuromuscular disease. Animals with spinal cord or neuromuscular disease do not have other signs suggestive of vestibular disease and do have signs attributable to their underlying problem, such as nonambulatory paresis. Animals with righting reaction deficits due to vestibular disease usually will have asymmetrical deficits; that is, they will try to rise from lateral recumbency on one side but not from the other side.

CLINICAL TIPS

- In animals with a head tilt, make sure to examine the eyes for strabismus and abnormal nystagmus when the animal is upright, lying on each side, and in dorsal recumbency.

- Subtle head tilts may become more obvious when the patient is blindfolded. Blindfolding eliminates visual input that helps compensate for vestibular dysfunction.

- Schiff-Sherrington syndrome is not necessarily a poor prognostic sign.

5

The Cranial Nerves

There are twelve pairs of cranial nerves (CNs) that innervate the structures of the head. All originate from the midbrain or medulla oblongata, except CNs I and II. One of each pair emerges from the left and right sides of the brain stem and innervates structures on the same side of the head. The central control of these nerves, whether it is motor control in the case of motor nerves or conscious perception of sensation in the case of the sensory nerves, is in the opposite cerebral cortex. This arrangement is important to remember when examining animals that have deficits in CN function secondary to higher center dysfunction. The CNs can be examined in any order, but carrying out the examination in numerical order of the nerves helps to ensure that the examiner will not overlook any part of the examination.

CRANIAL NERVE I: OLFACTORY NERVE

Function: The olfactory nerve is responsible for the sense of smell.

NEUROLOGICAL EXAMINATION

- Olfaction can be tested using any substance with an odor likely to attract the animal, such as a strong-smelling food (e.g., canned dog or cat food, fish, fresh meat, etc.). Cover the animal's eyes, or blindfold him, and bring the food substance close to his nose and move the food from side to side.

NORMAL FINDINGS

- The animal sniffs at the food, moving his nose closer to it, and follows the movement of the food by moving his head.

- Occasionally, the patient may dislike the odor presented. In that case, he should sniff at it, then move the head and neck away from it.

ABNORMAL FINDINGS

- The animal ignores the food and shows identical lack of reaction to several different types of odor.

CLINICAL NEUROANATOMY

- The olfactory nerve is a tract of the brain, rather than a true peripheral nerve.

- Receptors in the mucosa of the nasal passages are sensitive to chemical stimuli. The axons of these receptors travel back though the cribriform plate into the olfactory bulbs, the most rostral extensions of the cerebrum.

- The axons of the nasal sensory receptors synapse with secondary neurons in the olfactory bulbs. The axons of these secondary neurons project via several pathways to some of the most primitive parts of the forebrain, including the limbic system (responsible for emotions and many types of behavior), the reticular system, vomiting centers in the brain stem, and the cerebral cortex, where the sensory input reaches the level of consciousness and is recognized as smell.

CLINICAL TIPS

- Do not use volatile compounds such as ammonia to test sense of smell. These substances are noxious and stimulate receptors in the nasal cavity innervated by CN V, rather than those innervated by CN I.

- If the patient ignores the first stimulus, try one or two others; for example, use a meat foodstuff and then a fish-based foodstuff or a sweet odor.

- Animals that are very anxious may ignore olfactory stimuli. If you suspect that this is the problem with a patient, try repeating the test during a time and in an environment where the animal is more relaxed.

- Loss of the sense of smell is very rarely a consequence of primary neurological disease and is most commonly a result of disease in the nasal area. Apparent loss of sense of smell should prompt a thorough investigation of the nasal cavities for the presence of disease before it is determined to be a sign of primary neurological disease.

- Because loss of sense of smell is rarely due to primary neurological disease, testing an animal's sense of smell may not be considered an essential part of the neurological examination.

CRANIAL NERVE II: OPTIC NERVE

Function: The optic nerve is responsible for vision.

NEUROLOGICAL EXAMINATION

- Vision is tested most commonly by eliciting the menace reflex. Cover one of the animal's eyes with your hand. It is often convenient to slip the thumb of the same hand between the horizontal rami of the mandible, so as to keep the head up and stop the animal from pulling his head away. Open your other hand and face the palm toward the uncovered eye, about twelve inches away from the face (Figure 1). Make a sharp movement of your open palm toward the animal's right eye. The excursion of the movement should be three to four inches toward the animal's head.

- A second technique for testing vision is to move an object that the animal will follow. Have the animal sit or stand still, and when you have his attention, drop a cotton ball from

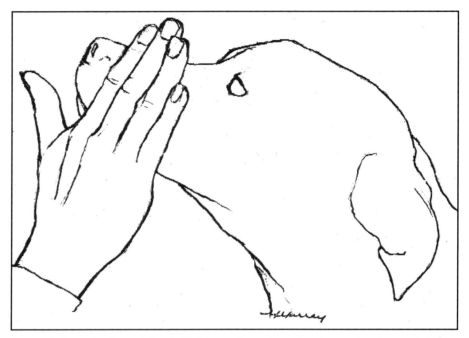

Figure 1. Examination of the Optic Nerve. *Face the palm of your hand toward the uncovered eye, about twelve inches away from the face.*

just above his head, twelve to eighteen inches in front of the face. A cotton ball produces almost no disturbance of the air and shows up well against most backgrounds.

- Vision can also be tested by setting up a maze. Simply permitting the animal to explore the unfamiliar environment of the examination room may be sufficient, or you may wish to place additional obstacles, such as boxes or chairs, in the room. This situation permits the testing of vision in different light conditions.

- Vision is evaluated when testing visual placing. Details of this test are described on page 82 in the chapter "Proprioception and the Postural Reactions."

NORMAL FINDINGS

- The normal response to the menace test is for the animal to blink the eye.

- Retraction of the globe, flicking of the third eyelid across the eye, and retraction of the head away from the threatening stimulus also may be observed.

- Most animals with normal sight will follow the path of a cotton ball dropped a short distance in front of the face by moving both the globes and the head in the direction of the cotton ball's path. If animals are distracted by surrounding noise or activity, it may take several attempts to attract the animal's attention.

- Animals should be able to negotiate around objects placed on the floor of the examination room.

ABNORMAL FINDINGS

- Animals that are blind will not blink in response to the menace test, may walk into objects placed in their path, and will not follow a cotton ball dropped close to the face.

CLINICAL NEUROANATOMY

- Sensory information from the retina travels in the optic nerve to the optic chiasm.

- In dogs and cats, 65% to 70% of the axons in the optic nerve cross the midline at the optic chiasm and ascend in the optic tract on the opposite side of the brain. Fibers that originate in the nasal part of the retina tend to cross at the optic chiasm, whereas those originating in the temporal part of the retina tend to remain ipsilateral.

- The crossing of some, but not all, optic nerve fibers at the optic chiasm accounts for the overlap of left and right visual field. Overlap is about 50% in cats and dogs. This makes it clear why the eye not being tested should be covered when eliciting the menace reflex.

- The majority of optic tract fibers synapse in the lateral geniculate body of the midbrain. Fibers from the lateral geniculate body then travel in the internal capsule to the occipital part of the cerebral cortex, where the sensory information is consciously perceived as vision. This is the principal but not the only pathway for vision.

- Output from the occipital cortex projects to the motor cortex and then ultimately to the nucleus of the facial nerve in the medulla. Motor activity in the facial nucleus causes blinking of the eye. Output from the motor cortex of the cerebrum onto other motor nuclei in the brain stem (particularly in the midbrain) results in the pull of the head away from the menace stimulus.

- Input from the cerebellum also plays a role in the menace reflex, although the exact pathway by which this occurs is unknown.

- Absence of the menace reflex may be due to a lesion resulting in blindness anywhere in the ascending visual pathway. Affected animals cannot negotiate a maze if blindness is bilateral; or if blindless is unilateral, they cannot negotiate a maze when the normal eye is blindfolded. Similarly, they will not track the path of a falling object. They can blink in response to tactile stimulation of the eye or face.

- Absence of the menace response also may be the result of facial nerve (CN VII) paralysis. In this case animals will pull away from a hand moved sharply toward the head, but they will not blink. They can negotiate a maze and will watch a cotton ball dropped just in front of the face. They will not blink in response to tactile stimulation of the eye or face, and they will have other signs of facial paralysis, such as drooping of the lips and ear on the affected side.

- Cerebellar disease may result in loss of the menace reflex. Animals can see and are able to blink, but they do not do so in response to the menace test. Other signs of cerebellar disease, such as intention tremor and hypermetria, are present.

- Because higher control of the motor arm of the reflex originates in the frontal lobe of the cerebral cortex, lesions here sometimes cause loss of the menace reflex, even in animals that have adequate vision.

CLINICAL TIPS

- A thorough ophthalmological examination is indicated in all cases where visual deficit or blindness is suspected, to help differentiate primary ocular from primary neurological causes of blindness.

- Decreased vision in moderate to low light conditions suggests primary ocular, rather than neurological, disease.

- It is essential not to touch the animal's face, eyelashes, or whiskers when eliciting the menace reflex. This will elicit a blink in response to the sensation of touch (sensory arm: CN V; motor arm: CN VII) rather than a blink in response to a visual stimulus.

- Some authors warn that even air movement may elicit a blink response, due to the movement of facial hairs caused by the air movement. It is this author's experience, however, that even vigorous hand movements close to the face will not produce a blink in animals that are truly blind, as long as the face, eyelashes, and whiskers are not touched.

- Moving a hand vertically just in front of the eye will elicit a blink response from most sighted animals, and this produces less air movement toward the face.

- Very anxious or excited animals or those that are dull or in a postictal state may not have a menace response and may ignore a dropped cotton ball, even when they have adequate vision. If you suspect this to be the case, recheck the menace response at a later time, when the animal's mental status is more normal.

CRANIAL NERVE III: OCULOMOTOR NERVE

Functions: The oculomotor nerve is responsible for movement of the globes and constriction of the pupils.

- The oculomotor nerve contains both a somatic component that innervates most of the extraocular muscles that move the globe and a parasympathetic component that innervates the circular muscle of the iris.

- Contraction of this muscle constricts the pupil.

- The somatic component of CN III innervates the extraocular muscles, except the lateral rectus, retractor bulbi, and dorsal oblique muscles.

- The functions of the somatic part of the oculomotor nerve are to maintain the globe in a central position in the orbit at rest and to move the globe appropriately when the head moves.

NEUROLOGICAL EXAMINATION

- **Oculocephalic reflex**
  — Observe the position of each eye within the orbit.
  — The somatic component of the oculomotor nerve is also tested by eliciting the oculocephalic reflex (i.e., physiological nystagmus). Turn the animal's head from side to side and observe the movement of the globes.

- **Pupillary light reflex**
  — Eliciting the pupillary light reflex tests the parasympathetic component of CN III. Shine a bright light into the eye being tested (Figure 2). Different parts of the visual field can be tested by shining the light first from the lateral aspect onto the nasal part of the retina, then from the medial aspect onto the temporal part of the retina.

NORMAL FINDINGS

- The normal position of the globe is central within the orbit. The patient should be able to move both globes to track moving objects or in response to visual or auditory stimuli (i.e., moving the eyes to see an object at the edge of the visual field or in response to a noise from one side).

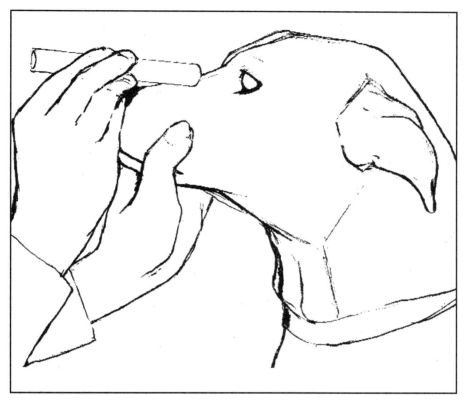

Figure 2. Eliciting the Pupillary Light Reflex. *Shine a bright light into the eye being tested.*

- When the head is turned from side to side, the normal response is a horizontal nystagmus with the fast phase of the movement toward the direction of the movement of the head. The reflex can be thought of as the globe "catching up" with the movement of the head. A similar but vertical nystagmus is observed when the head is moved up and down in a "nodding" motion. Most animals, however, resent the rapid extension and flexion of the head needed to elicit an obvious vertical nystagmus. If the position of the globes at rest, the voluntary movements of the globes, and the oculocephalic reflex when the head is moved from side to side all are normal, it is not necessary to test the oculo-cephalic reflex in response to vertical movement of the head.

- The normal pupillary light reflex is constriction of the pupil in the eye being tested (direct response). The pupil in the opposite eye also constricts (indirect response).

ABNORMAL FINDINGS

- Paralysis of the somatic component of the oculomotor nerve causes a ventrolateral strabismus of the globe. The strabismus is constant in all positions of the head and body. The oculocephalic reflex is abolished, and the patient cannot voluntarily move the globe.

- Paralysis of the parasympathetic component of the nerve results in a dilated pupil in the affected eye, which is unresponsive even to bright light. When light shines into the affected eye, the animal may blink or try to avert the head, because the visual pathway is normal, but the pupil will not constrict (abnormal direct response). The pupil in the opposite, normal eye constricts (normal indirect response). When a light shines into the opposite, normal eye, that pupil will constrict (normal direct response); the pupil in the affected eye will not constrict (abnormal indirect response). Lesions of the visual system are summarized in Table 5.

CLINICAL NEUROANATOMY

- The sensory modality for the oculocephalic reflex is not visual but vestibular. Angular movement of the head is detected by the receptors in the three semicircular canals of the inner ear. Information from the semicircular canal receptors passes, via the vestibular ganglion and CN VIII, to the vestibular nuclei in the medulla and vestibular system elements in the cerebellum. Axons then project rostrally in a pathway called the medial longitudinal fasciculus (MLF) to the somatic nucleus of CN III in the midbrain, the nucleus of CN IV (also located in the midbrain), and the nucleus of CN VI in the rostral medulla. Vestibular input directs activity in these three CNs, maintaining conjugate movements of both eyes and the normal position of the globes within the orbits.

TABLE 5

Location of Lesions Causing Visual and Ocular Abnormalities[1]

Lesion Location	Vision		Menace Response		Pupil Size[2]		Direct PLR[3]		Indirect PLR[4]		Comments
	L Eye	R Eye	L Eye	R Eye	L Eye	R Eye	L Eye	R Eye	L Eye	R Eye	
Left retina or optic nerve	Absent	Normal	Absent	Normal	Normal to slight dilatation	Normal	Absent	Normal	Absent	Normal	Perform a thorough ophthalmic examination
Right retina or optic nerve	Normal	Absent	Normal	Absent	Normal	Normal to slight dilatation	Normal	Absent	Normal	Absent	
Optic chiasma (complete, bilateral) or both retinae, or both optic nerves	Absent	Absent	Absent	Widely dilated	Widely dilated	Absent	Absent	Absent	Absent	Absent	
Left optic tract	Normal to slightly decreased	Decreased	Normal to slightly decreased	Decreased to absent	Normal to slight miosis	Normal to slight dilatation	Normal	Reduced	Reduced	Normal	Lesions of the optic tracts are difficult to distinguish from lesions affecting the ipsilateral cerebral hemispheres

TABLE 5 (continued)

Location of Lesions Causing Visual and Ocular Abnormalities[1]

Lesion Location	Vision		Menace Response		Pupil Size[2]		Direct PLR[3]		Indirect PLR[4]		Comments
	L Eye	R Eye	L Eye	R Eye	L Eye	R Eye	L Eye	R Eye	L Eye	R Eye	
Right optic tract	Decreased	Normal to slightly decreased	Decreased to absent	Normal to slightly decreased	Normal to slight dilatation	Normal to slight miosis	Reduced	Normal	Reduced	Normal	(See Left optic tract)
Left midbrain[5]	Normal	Normal	Normal	Normal	Dilated	Normal	Absent	Normal	Normal	Absent	Animals with midbrain disease usually have ARAS[6] involvement and severe changes in consciousness
Right midbrain[5]	Normal	Normal	Normal	Normal	Normal	Dilated	Normal	Absent	Absent	Normal	
Left cerebrum	Normal	Absent	Normal	Absent	Normal	Normal	Normal	Normal	Normal	Normal	Animals with cerebral disease often have other signs such as circling, seizures, and decreased consciousness
Right cerebrum	Absent	Normal	Absent	Normal	Normal	Normal	Normal	Normal	Normal	Normal	

TABLE 5 (continued)
Location of Lesions Causing Visual and Ocular Abnormalities[1]

Lesion Location	Vision		Menace Response		Pupil Size[2]		Direct PLR[3]		Indirect PLR[4]		Comments
	L Eye	R Eye	L Eye	R Eye	L Eye	R Eye	L Eye	R Eye	L Eye	R Eye	
Left Horner's syndrome (sympathetic)	Normal	Normal	Normal	Normal	Small (miotic)	Normal	Normal (may be hard to detect if pupil very miotic)	Normal	Normal (may be hard to detect if pupil very miotic)	Normal	Look for other signs of Horner's syndrome, such as ptosis, enophthalmos, and protrusion of the third eyelid in the affected eye
Right Horner's syndrome	Normal	Normal	Normal	Normal	Normal	Small (miotic)	Normal	Normal (may be hard to detect if pupil very miotic)	Normal	Normal (may be hard to detect if pupil very miotic)	

1 The descriptions in this table refer to lesions that are complete or, at least, severe. Partial lesions cause lesser abnormalities; for example, a partial retinal lesion may cause decreased vision and reduced direct pupillary light reflex in the affected eye, rather than blindness and absense of direct pupillary light reflex.
2 Pupil size refers to size of the pupils when both eyes are illuminated equally in normal ambient light (i.e., daylight).
3 PLR = pupillary light response
4 Indirect PLR: The left indirect PLR is the response seen in the right pupil when light is shone in the left eye. The right indirect PLR is the response seen in the left pupil when light is shone in the right eye.
5 Lesions affecting the midbrain are most often bilateral rather than lateralized. Animals with facial paresis or paralysis (CN VII) have reduced to absent menace response on the affected side, but normal visual responses otherwise. Animals with cerebellar lesions may lack menace response on the affected side, or bilaterally, but have normal visual responses otherwise. Animals that are excited or anxious often have reduced menace response and pupillary responses bilaterally but have normal vision, and return to normal once they become less excited or anxious.
6 ARAS = Ascending Reticular Activating System

Vision does not play a role in this pathway, so animals that are blind but have no other brain dysfunction have normal position of the globes and normal oculocephalic reflexes.

- The distal part of the sensory arm of the pupillary light reflex is identical to that for vision and the menace reflex. Sensory fibers pass from the retina, via the optic nerve and optic chiasm, to the optic tract. A small number of optic tract fibers project to the pretectal nucleus in the midbrain. Eighty percent of fibers from the pretectal nucleus cross the midline and project to the parasympathetic nucleus of the oculomotor nerve, which also is in the midbrain. Visual input thus reaches the origin of the parasympathetic nerve supply to the eye. It should be noted that this pathway crosses the midline twice: once at the optic chiasm and once after exiting the pretectal nucleus. Shining a light into one eye, therefore, ultimately results in constriction of the pupil of the same eye. Some of the fibers originating in the pretectal nucleus do not cross the midline but project to the ipsilateral parasympathetic nucleus of the oculomotor nerve. Activity in this pathway accounts for the indirect pupillary light reflex.

- Globe position, conjugate movements of the eyes, and oculocephalic reflexes may be abnormal when lesions are present in the vestibular system or in CNs III, IV, or VI. The latter two are discussed below. In severe disease affecting the midbrain, which is a common result of traumatic brain injury, the pupils are dilated and nonresponsive to light, the oculocephalic reflexes are absent, and ventrolateral strabismus may be present. Coma and decerebrate posture usually accompany these ocular signs. Animals with this constellation of clinical signs have a guarded to poor prognosis.

- The axons of the oculomotor nerve travel forward along the floor of the cranial vault to the orbital fissure, where they exit into the orbit and thence to their terminations in the extraocular muscles (somatic component) and the pupillary constrictor muscle (parasympathetic component). Thus, lesions in the midbrain, on the floor of the cranium, or in the orbit may involve the oculomotor nerve.

CLINICAL TIPS

- Use a bright light when testing the pupillary light reflex.

- Reducing the ambient light level slightly may facilitate observation of a brisk pupillary light reflex.

- Animals that are excited or anxious may have moderately dilated pupils due to sympathetic nervous system activation. When the pupillary light reflex is tested in such cases, the response should be brisk; but the pupil may not constrict as completely as expected. Retest the patient when he is calmer.

- It may be helpful to have an assistant watch for the indirect pupillary light reflex while the examiner watches for the direct reflex.

- The pupillary light reflex may be difficult to observe in animals with very dark iris color. The following technique may help. Reduce the ambient light level to quite low. Stand about three to four feet away from the patient, with his head facing you. Look through a direct ophthalmoscope at the patient's face; you should be able to see a bright reflection from both retinas. Now test or have an assistant test the pupillary light reflex. Constriction of the pupil should be easy to observe as the shrinking of the area of tapetal reflection.

CRANIAL NERVE IV: TROCHLEAR NERVE

Function: The trochlear nerve is responsible for medial rotation of the dorsal aspect of the globe.

NEUROLOGICAL EXAMINATION

- Observe the orientation of the globe within the orbit. A fundic examination to observe the orientation of the retinal vasculature is necessary in dogs.

NORMAL FINDINGS

- The orientation of the pupil in cats is vertical. The dorsal (i.e., superior) retinal vein is oriented vertically in cats and dogs and can be seen when the fundus is examined with an ophthalmoscope.

ABNORMAL FINDINGS

- The pupil in cats and the dorsal retinal vein in both cats and dogs are deviated, with the dorsal aspect of each directed more laterally than normal. The dog has a round pupil; therefore, abnormalities of globe orientation secondary to trochlear nerve dysfunction can be appreciated only by examining the retina.

CLINICAL NEUROANATOMY

- The cell bodies of the neurons that form the trochlear nerve are located in a nucleus in the ventral midbrain. After crossing the midline twice, close to their origin, the axons of trochlear neurons travel rostrally along the floor of the cranial vault and exit the skull through the orbital fissure, along with CNs III and VI. Lesions of the midbrain, on the floor of the cranial vault, or in the orbit may involve the trochlear nerve.

CLINICAL TIPS

- Perform a fundic examination in animals to determine the orientation of the retinal vasculature.

- Trochlear nerve lesions are rare and are almost certain to be accompanied by signs of problems in adjacent structures, such as evidence of midbrain disease or lesions of CN III or VI.

CRANIAL NERVE VI: ABDUCENT NERVE

Function: The abducent nerve is responsible for lateral movement of the globes and retraction of the globes. The abducent nerve is discussed here because it is the third nerve involved in control of globe position and movements.

NEUROLOGICAL EXAMINATION

- Observe the position of the globes within the orbits and the voluntary movements of the eyes.

- Test the oculocephalic reflex as described previously (see Cranial nerve III).

- Dampen the tip of a cotton swab with water. Holding the eyelids open, gently touch the surface of the central cornea (Figure 3).

NORMAL FINDINGS

- The globes should be central within the orbits, and a full range of voluntary eye movements should be present.

- Normal oculocephalic reflexes should be elicited (see Cranial nerve III).

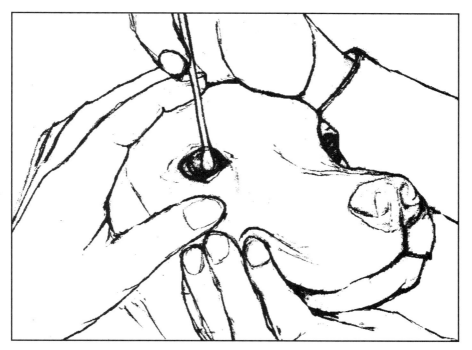

Figure 3. Examination of the Abducent Nerve. *Holding the eyelids open, gently touch the surface of the central cornea.*

- When the surface of the cornea is touched, the globe should be withdrawn into the orbit, the third eyelid should protrude across the cornea, and the animal should attempt to close the eyelids.

ABNORMAL FINDINGS

- Abducent nerve lesions cause paralysis of the lateral rectus muscle. The globe cannot be moved laterally, and medial strabismus is present.

- Medial deviation of the globes is maintained when testing physiological nystagmus.

- Although the patient retracts his head and attempts to close his eyes when the surface of the cornea is touched, the globe cannot be retracted into the orbit and the third eyelid does not protrude completely across the surface of the cornea.

CLINICAL NEUROANATOMY

- The cell bodies of the abducent neurons lie in the rostral medulla oblongata.

- The nerve courses rostrally along the floor of the cranial vault, exiting through the orbital fissure along with CNs II and IV.

- The abducent nerve may be damaged within the rostral medulla, as it passes along the floor of the cranial vault, or in the orbit.

- The sensory innervation of the cornea is via CN V, described below. Lesions in this nerve may abolish the retractor bulbi reflex, but globe position and oculocephalic reflexes are normal.

CLINICAL TIPS

- Lesions of CN VI are rare and would be expected to be accompanied by signs of damage to adjacent structures in the medulla or in CNs III and IV.

- Inability to retract the globe is commonly a result of retro-bulbar lesions. A complete ophthalmological examination should be carried out in animals that are unable to retract the globe.

- An abscess or tumor in a retrobulbar location may be a source of pain, so the animal may cry when the retractor bulbi reflex is elicited.

SYMPATHETIC INNERVATION TO THE EYE

No discussion of neurological causes of ocular abnormality would be complete without mentioning the sympathetic innervation to the eye.

Function: The sympathetic innervation to the eye is responsible for dilation of the pupil, retraction of the third eyelid, retraction of the upper eyelid, and rostral protrusion of the globe.

NEUROLOGICAL EXAMINATION

- Observe the structures of the eye, including the position of the third eyelid, the width of the palpebral aperture, and the size of the pupil.

NORMAL FINDINGS

- The position of the third eyelid, the width of the palpebral aperture, and the size of the pupil are all within normal parameters, and there is symmetry between the two eyes.

ABNORMAL FINDINGS

- Damage to the sympathetic innervation of the eye causes Horner's syndrome, with the following constellation of clinical signs.
  — Ptosis: Drooping of the upper eyelid due to denervation of the *levator palpebrae superioris* muscle.
  — Miosis: Mild to moderate constriction of the pupil due to denervation of the radial muscle of the iris.

— Enophthalmos: Sinking of the globe into the orbit due to denervation of smooth muscle in the orbit, which normally pushes the globe rostrally.

— Protrusion of the third eyelid: Caused by denervation of the retractor muscle of the third eyelid.

CLINICAL NEUROANATOMY

• The upper motor neurons of the sympathetic innervation to the eye originate in the midbrain.

• Axons travel down the cervical spinal cord in the tecto-tegmentospinal tract and synapse on preganglionic sympathetic neurons in spinal cord segments T_1-T_3.

• The axons of the preganglionic sympathetic nerves emerge from the spinal canal, along with the spinal nerves that form the brachial plexus, and ascend the neck in the vagosympathetic trunk.

• The preganglionic sympathetic nerves synapse with postganglionic neurons in the cranial cervical ganglion medial to the lower jaw.

• The axons of the postganglionic sympathetic neurons course rostrally with the carotid artery, passing close to the petrous temporal bone and the wall of the middle ear.

• These axons subsequently pass alongside the ophthalmic branch of the trigeminal nerve into the orbit and thence to the globe.

CLINICAL TIPS

• Horner's syndrome can result from lesions anywhere along the sympathetic pathway described previously.

• Lesions causing Horner's syndrome can be localized to pre- or postganglionic lesions, using pharmacological testing. One drop of 2.5% phenylephrine instilled into the eye will result in mydriasis within 20 minutes in an eye affected by a postganglionic sympathetic nerve lesion. In a normal eye or an eye affected by a preganglionic sympathetic nerve lesion, dilation either will not occur or will take 30-45 minutes.

- When anisocoria is present *and no primary ocular lesions are found*, a quick way of determining its cause is as follows. Place the animal in darkness for a few minutes and then observe the pupil size using a dim light. If both pupils dilate to equal size, the sympathetic innervation to both eyes is normal. The pupil that is more dilated is abnormal, due to a lesion affecting the oculomotor nerve. If the pupils do not dilate to equality, the eye with the smaller pupil is abnormal, which is caused by Horner's syndrome.

CRANIAL NERVE V: TRIGEMINAL NERVE

Functions: The trigeminal nerve provides proprioceptive and tactile sensory innervation to the face and head, including the eyes and mouth. The mandibular branch of the nerve supplies motor innervation to the masticatory muscles.

NEUROLOGICAL EXAMINATION

- Use the tip of a closed hemostat to touch the nares (Figure 4). Touch the periorbital area with your fingers (Figure 5). Again use the hemostat to touch the brow, the nose (Figure 6), the cheeks, and the lower jaw (Figure 7).

- Observe and palpate the temporalis and masseter muscles on each side of the head.

- Open the jaw and test the amount of muscular resistance (i.e., jaw tone).

- Observe the animal eating.

NORMAL FINDINGS

- When the face is touched, the animal should try to avert or retract the head; he will blink (especially when the periorbital area is stimulated); and he may wrinkle the upper lip.

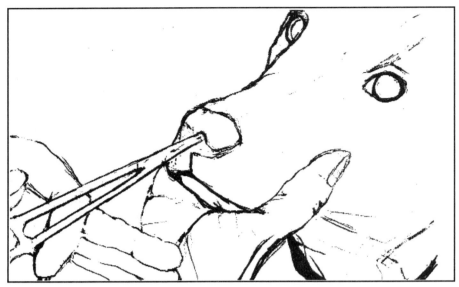

Figure 4. Examination of the Trigeminal Nerve. *Touch the nares.*

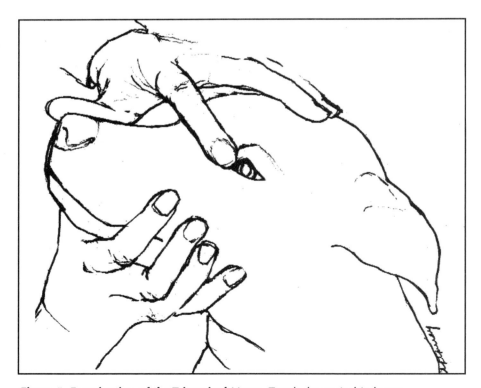

Figure 5. Examination of the Trigeminal Nerve. *Touch the periorbital area.*

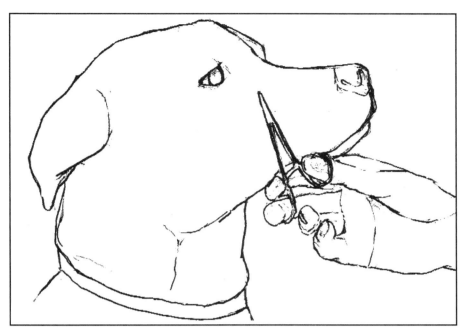

Figure 6. Examination of the Trigeminal Nerve. *Touch the nose.*

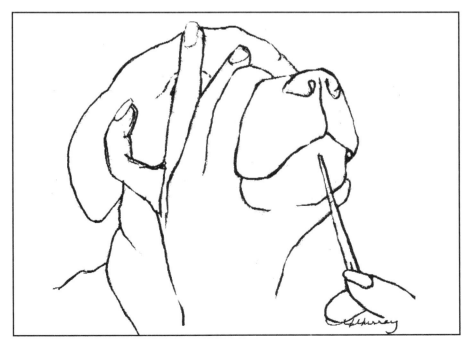

Figure 7. Examination of the Trigeminal Nerve. *Touch the the lower jaw.*

- The temporalis and masseter muscles mass should be normal for that size and type of animal and be bilaterally symmetrical.

- There should be moderate resistance on opening the mouth.

- Prehension and eating, particularly chewing, should be normal.

ABNORMAL FINDINGS

- Animals with lesions of the sensory components of the trigeminal nerve will have reduced or absent sensation over the face and head.

- If only a single branch of the nerve is involved, sensory loss will involve only local areas of the face and head.

- Lesions of the motor component of the trigeminal nerve result in atrophy of the temporalis and masseter muscles.

- Jaw tone is decreased when lesions of the motor component of CN V are present.

- Bilateral motor involvement of CN V causes a dropped lower jaw. The animal is unable to close his mouth and has great difficulty eating and drinking.

CLINICAL NEUROANATOMY

- The cell bodies of the sensory neurons in the trigeminal nerve lie in a ganglion within the cranial vault, in the area of the petrous temporal bone. The axons of these sensory neurons project distally as the ophthalmic, maxillary, and mandibular branches of CN V.

- The ophthalmic branch transmits sensory information from the globe, the forehead, and part of the periorbital area. The maxillary branch transmits sensory information from the foreface, part of the periorbital area, the nares, and part of the mouth. The mandibular branch transmits sensory information from the lower jaw area and part of the mouth.

- Ascending input from the sensory components of CN V projects to a long chain of sensory nuclei that extend the length of the medulla oblongata, caudally into the rostral portion of the cervical spinal cord, and rostrally into the caudal midbrain. Information is relayed from these centers to the brain stem motor centers that control reflex responses, such as blinking, and to the cerebral cortex, reaching the level of conscious perception.

- The motor neuron cell bodies, whose axons travel in the mandibular branch of CN V, are located in the pons. These neurons innervate the muscles of mastication, including the masseter, temporalis, pterygoid, and digastricus muscles. The first two are the most easily examined.

- Lesions of the motor component of the trigeminal nerve may be either central or peripheral in location. In the former case, CNS structures close to the pons may also be affected, including CNs VII and VIII, the vestibular system, long motor and sensory tracts to the limbs, and the cerebellum.

- Sensory deficits due to trigeminal nerve lesions are almost certainly peripheral in location. The central sensory component of CN V is so large (extending from the midbrain to the rostral cervical spinal cord) that lesions extensive enough to destroy this whole pathway will likely be fatal.

- The motor component of the reflex pathway for facial sensation is effected mostly through the facial nerve, CN VII.

CLINICAL TIPS

- A light, tactile stimulus to the face is often adequate to elicit an obvious reflex response.

- If light touch is not effective, other stimuli can be used, such as a skin pinch with a hemostat or a pinprick. Use caution around the eyes.

- The sensory arm of the corneal reflex (described previously in the discussion of CN VI functions) involves the trigeminal nerve.

- In the dog, the lateral canthus area receives sensory innervation from the maxillary nerve alone, while the medial canthus area and the cornea receive sensory innervation from the ophthalmic nerve alone. In the cat, only the cornea receives sensory innervation from the ophthalmic nerve alone.

- The lower jaw is not particularly sensitive. Stimulating the chin may produce little response, even in a normal animal. The lower lip, which also receives sensory innervation from the mandibular nerve, is very sensitive. Lightly touching the lower lip will usually produce a quick retraction of the head in a normal animal.

- Animals with cerebral lesions may appear to have reduced sensory function on the contralateral side of the face. This can be mistaken for a lesion of the sensory components of CN V. With cerebral lesions, the animal will be dull and have other signs of cerebral disease, such as ipsiversive circling and contralateral postural reaction deficits. Animals with lateralized central lesions of the sensory component of CN V may also be dull, and they may circle. These animals usually have ipsilateral hemiparesis as well as postural deficits, and they circle toward, rather than away from, the side of the limb paresis.

- Unilateral lesions of the mandibular nerve cause atrophy of the masticatory muscles on one side, but weakness of the jaw usually is not obvious or is mild.

- Many normal animals have been taught to open the mouth readily, therefore, jaw tone may not be appreciated accurately.

- Bilateral lesions of the mandibular nerve cause atrophy of the masticatory muscles bilaterally, weakness of the jaw, and a jaw drop.

- Animals with primary disease of the masticatory muscles have atrophy of the affected muscles, which is usually bilateral. The jaw is not dropped, however, but is often difficult or impossible to open because of muscle atrophy and fibrosis.

- Rabies is an important differential diagnosis in animals with a dropped jaw.

- Inability to close the mouth when bilateral mandibular nerve disease is present may result in difficulty eating and drinking, drooling of saliva, and dehydration if fluid balance is not maintained.

- Older animals of some breeds, particularly the dolichocephalic breeds like the Doberman pinscher and the greyhound, often have decreased temporal muscle mass without obvious signs of clinical dysfunction. The cause and significance of this finding are unknown.

CRANIAL NERVE VII : FACIAL NERVE

Functions: The facial nerve serves as the motor to the muscles of facial expression. It transmits the sensation of taste from the rostral two-thirds of the tongue, transmits tactile sensory information from the medial aspect of the pinna, and promotes salivation and lacrimation via its parasympathetic component.

NEUROLOGICAL EXAMINATION

- Observe the face for symmetry of facial musculature and normal facial movements during eating, drinking, barking, etc.

- The motor function of CN VII is examined when testing for the presence of facial sensation and the corneal reflex, and when performing the menace test (all described previously).

- Stroke the medial aspect of the pinna with the tip of a closed hemostat (Figure 8).

- Lacrimation can be measured using the Schirmer tear test.

- Other functions of CN VII, such as the sensation of taste and production of saliva, are generally not tested during a routine neurological examination.

NORMAL FINDINGS

- The facial musculature is symmetrical.

- The facial muscles move and the animal blinks when the face is stimulated with a tactile stimulus, such as a hemostat tip, or when the corneal reflex is tested.

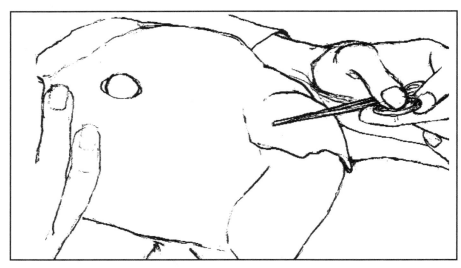

Figure 8. Examination of the Facial Nerve. *Stroke the medial aspect of the pinna with the tip of a closed hemostat.*

- The animal blinks in response to the menace test.

- Touching the medial aspect of the pinna of the ear causes a reflex twitch of the ear.

ABNORMAL FINDINGS

- Acute unilateral facial nerve paresis to paralysis causes drooping of the face on one side, most noticeable in the lip and ear. The nose is pulled slightly toward the normal side.

- In chronic facial nerve lesions, drooping of the lip may be less obvious and the nose may be pulled toward the abnormal side because of atrophy and contracture of the facial muscles on that side.

- The animal may drool from the affected side of the mouth.

- When the face is stimulated, the animal may pull his head away, because the sensation of touch (transmitted by branches of CN V) is still perceived; however, he cannot blink or wrinkle the lip.

- The ear does not move when the medial pinna is touched.

CLINICAL NEUROANATOMY

- The cell bodies of the motor neurons of CN VII lie within a nucleus in the rostral medulla and caudal midbrain.

- The cell bodies of the sensory neurons of CN VII lie in the geniculate ganglion, within the petrous temporal bone. Central projections of these cells terminate mainly in the medulla oblongata. Information is then relayed to a variety of brain-stem nuclei for reflex responses and to the cerebral cortex for conscious recognition of taste and tactile stimuli.

- The motor, sensory, and parasympathetic components of CN VII run together for only a short distance, from just within the cranial vault to shortly after the nerve exits the skull in the vicinity of the petrous temporal bone. Only when lesions occur in this area will motor, sensory, and parasympathetic deficits occur in combination. Peripheral lesions of CN VII tend to cause only facial paresis to paralysis.

- Lesions of the parasympathetic component of CN VII cause decreased tear production (i.e., keratoconjunctivitis sicca).

- The sensory branches of CN VII to the medial pinna contain some fibers from the vagus nerve that join and are distributed with the fibers of CN VII. This is of little clinical importance.

CRANIAL NERVE VIII: VESTIBULOCOCHLEAR NERVE

Function: The vestibulocochlear nerve is responsible for hearing and position sense (i.e., vestibular function).

NEUROLOGICAL EXAMINATION

- Observe the patient's response to noise.

- With the animal facing away from the owner, have the owner call the animal's name or make a loud noise behind the animal.

- Observe the animal for head tilt, circling, spontaneous nystagmus, or strabismus.

- Place the animal in lateral recumbency on each side and in dorsal recumbency, and observe for spontaneous nystagmus or strabismus.

- Test the oculocephalic reflexes (as described on page 36).

NORMAL FINDINGS

- The animal turns toward sounds made behind him or to one side.

- Head tilt and spontaneous nystagmus are absent.

- The oculocephalic reflexes are normal (see page 37).

ABNORMAL FINDINGS

- The animal does not respond to sounds.

- In unilateral deafness, the animal may be alert but does not turn toward the sound, or he may turn in the wrong direction.

- Head tilt and spontaneous nystagmus are present (see Posture and Attitude chapter and Table 4).

- The oculocephalic reflex is absent or reduced. When the lesion is unilateral, the oculocephalic reflex usually is decreased when the head is turned toward the side of the lesion.

CLINICAL NEUROANATOMY

- Receptors both for the auditory and vestibular systems lie in the inner ear. The former lie within the cochlear apparatus, whereas the latter lie in the utricule (detecting craniocaudal acceleration of the head), the saccule (detecting vertical acceleration of the head), and the three semicircular canals (detecting angular acceleration of the head).

- Axons from both the vestibular and auditory receptors in the inner ear course toward the medulla in CN VIII, synapsing in the vestibular and cochlear nucleus, respectively. Central connections extend widely and bilaterally in both of these systems, both to brain-stem centers for reflex responses (such as the oculocephalic reflex) and to the cerebral cortex.

CLINICAL TIPS

- When testing hearing, ensure that sound is coming from only one source. A lot of noise from different directions may be confusing to the patient and he may not exhibit a clear response.

- Having the owner call the animal's name usually works very well. Otherwise use a sharp, loud sound, such as a whistle.

- It is impossible to accurately determine various levels of hearing loss in the examination room. Objective tests, such as brain-stem auditory-evoked responses, are required. These tests are beyond the scope of this discussion.

- "Selective deafness" caused by the animal's choosing to ignore the sound stimulus can be remarkable in animals. Again, objective testing is the only way to be certain of the status of the auditory system in animals.

- True deafness is most likely peripheral in origin, caused by lesions in the ear or CN VIII. Because the central projection of auditory input is bilateral and widespread within the brain, central lesions do not cause complete deafness unless they are very extensive and severe. In this case, numerous other signs of neurological disease will be present.

- When looking for spontaneous nystagmus, make sure to observe the animal for several seconds after changing the position of the head and body. Spontaneous nystagmus sometimes appears immediately after changing position, then disappears, or only appears when the animal has been in the new position for several seconds.

- Having the head in one position (e.g., with the nose facing the ceiling) and the body in another (e.g., laterally recumbent) may elicit spontaneous nystagmus in animals with subtle vestibular lesions.

- Subtle, spontaneous nystagmus may be superimposed on normal eye movements. Observing the animal for several seconds or longer will help to detect this.

CRANIAL NERVES IX AND X: VAGUS AND GLOSSOPHARYNGEAL

Functions: The vagus and glossopharyngeal nerves are responsible for motor and sensory innervation to the pharynx and larynx. The vagus nerve also provides parasympathetic innervation to the majority of the thoracic and abdominal viscera, as well as performing several other functions.

NEUROLOGICAL EXAMINATION

- Open the animal's mouth and test the gag reflex by placing a finger over the back of the tongue into the rostral part of the pharynx (Figure 9).

NORMAL FINDINGS

- The animal will gag, pushing the base of the tongue rostrally and dorsally, and will often make a retching sound.

ABNORMAL FNDINGS

- The animal may not object to a finger pushed into the pharynx, or he may try to escape from the stimulus, but he will not have a gag reflex.

- Laryngeal weakness may be apparent as stertorous breathing, especially during and after exercise.

CLINICAL NEUROANATOMY

- The motor fibers of CNs IX and X to the pharynx and larynx arise from the nucleus ambiguus, which extends through the middle and caudal medulla oblongata. The sensory fibers of both nerves have their cell bodies in the nucleus of the solitary tract, also in the medulla oblongata.

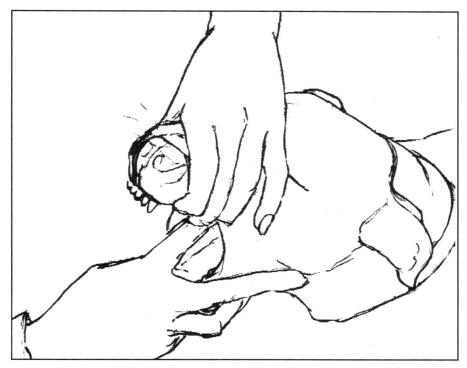

Figure 9. Examination of the Vagus and Glossopharyngeal Nerves. Test the gag reflex by placing a finger over the back of the tongue into the rostral part of the pharynx.

- Cranial nerves IX and X have numerous other functions that are not specifically tested during routine neurological examination.

- Lesions in the mid- to caudal medulla can cause loss of the gag reflex and laryngeal paralysis. Quadriparesis and ataxia usually accompany such lesions.

- Unilateral lesions of CNs IX and X usually do not cause obvious loss of the gag reflex, but laryngeal hemiplegia does cause stertor and possible exercise intolerance.

- Peripheral lesions in the vagus nerve, particularly in the recurrent laryngeal nerves, also cause laryngeal hemiplegia or paralysis.

CLINICAL TIPS

- If there is a risk of being bitten, do not test the gag reflex, but observe the animal eating and drinking. Functional deficits in the pharynx and larynx cause dysphagia, coughing, and gagging.

- Laryngeal paresis or paralysis may cause a change in bark or meow (i.e., dysphonia).

- Animals with pharyngeal and laryngeal weakness are at great risk of aspiration pneumonia, a life-threatening complication.

- Inflammation or mass lesions in the wall of the pharynx or larynx may cause signs that mimic pharyngeal and laryngeal paresis or paralysis.

- Diffuse lower motor neuron and neuromuscular diseases, such as botulism, myasthenia gravis, and hypothyroidism, also can cause laryngeal and pharyngeal dysfunction.

CRANIAL NERVE XI: ACCESSORY NERVE

Function: The accessory nerve is responsible for motor innervation of the brachiocephalic, sternocephalic, and trapezius muscles.

NEUROLOGICAL EXAMINATION

- Palpate the dorsal and lateral aspects of the neck and shoulder region.

NORMAL FINDINGS

- The musculature of the neck and shoulder has normal mass and tone and is symmetrical.

ABNORMAL FINDINGS

- Atrophy and asymmetry of the muscles innervated by CN XI occur.

CLINICAL NEUROANATOMY

- The cell bodies of the accessory nerve lie in the nucleus ambiguus in the mid- to caudal medulla oblongata, together with those of the vagus and glossopharyngeal nerves.

CLINICAL TIPS

- Lesions of the accessory nerve are extremely rare.

CRANIAL NERVE XII: HYPOGLOSSAL NERVE

Function: The hypoglossal nerve acts as a motor to the tongue.

NEUROLOGICAL EXAMINATION

- When testing the gag reflex (as described previously), examine the tongue for symmetry. The tongue also can be pulled from the mouth to appreciate its strength.

NORMAL FINDINGS

- The tongue is symmetrical, does not deviate to one side or the other, and can be moved freely.

- When pulled out of the mouth, the tongue retracts immediately when it is released.

ABNORMAL FINDINGS

- In acute unilateral lesions of the hypoglossal nerve, the tongue deviates toward the normal side. The muscular tone on the normal side is unopposed by the denervated muscle on the abnormal side.

- In chronic lesions, the abnormal side of the tongue atrophies and contracts. The tongue deviates toward the abnormal side.

CLINICAL NEUROANATOMY

- The cell bodies of the hypoglossal nerve lie in the hypoglossal nucleus in the caudal medulla oblongata. Medullary lesions affecting the hypoglossal nucleus also tend to cause ipsilateral hemiparesis and ataxia.

6

Gait and Movement

Gait and movement are observed before commencing the "hands on" parts of the neurological examination.

NORMAL FINDINGS

The animal should move around the room in a coordinated manner and be able to negotiate stairs and other small obstacles. Cats may not be asked to walk up and down stairs, but they may offer actions such as jumping onto and off furniture.

ABNORMAL FINDINGS

A wide variety of abnormalities may be observed in gait and movement.

Ataxia

- Ataxia is a swaying gait in one to four limbs that is the result of loss of position sense. The patient may stagger, adduct, or abduct the limbs excessively and appear to be "drunk." He may knuckle over onto the dorsum of the paws. Examine the toenails; ataxic animals often have scraped the dorsum of the paws and have obviously worn toenails. Animals may be unable to climb or descend stairs and are in danger of falling. Ataxia is usually accompanied by paresis.

Paresis

- Paresis is a descriptive term for weakness. The limbs may be held in a more flexed position than normal. The feet are not lifted normally and tend to drag on the ground when the animal walks. Animals may be unable to climb or descend stairs and are in danger of falling.

- Ataxia and paresis usually occur together and may be difficult to clearly distinguish in the patient; both contribute to gait abnormalities. In order of worsening severity of signs, gait can be classified as follows.
  — *Normal gait*
  — *Ambulatory paresis:* The patient can walk, but weakness (and usually ataxia) is present in the affected limbs. Weakness in all four limbs also is called quadriparesis or tetraparesis. Paresis of both limbs on one side of the body is called hemiparesis. Paresis of the hind limbs alone is called paraparesis.
  — *Nonambulatory paresis:* The patient is too weak and ataxic to bear weight, but voluntary movement is still present. Voluntary movement occurs without noxious stimuli applied to the affected limbs.
  — *Paralysis:* The patient cannot walk, and voluntary movement is absent. Reflex movement, such as withdrawal in response to a pinch of the toe, may still be present. Paralysis of all four limbs also is called quadriplegia or tetraplegia. Paralysis of both limbs on one side of the body is called hemiplegia. Paralysis of the hind limbs alone is called paraplegia.

- The severity of gait deficits may be symmetrical from side to side and between the fore- and hind limbs, or it may be asymmetrical. Remember that lesions in the brain rostral to the medulla oblongata cause contralateral abnormalities in gait, proprioception, and postural reactions. Abnormalities in the medulla, the cerebellum, the spinal cord, or peripheral nerves cause ipsilateral deficits.

Dysmetria, Hypermetria

- Loss of control of the range and force of movement is called dysmetria. It is most commonly evident as hypermetria. In hypermetria, the onset of movement in the limb is slightly delayed, and then the limb movement is excessive in range and force. This is evident as a "high-stepping gait." The foot may be slapped down rather hard at the end of the movement.

Tremor

- Tremor is another common abnormality of movement seen in animals with neurological disease. Tremor is caused by oscillating contraction of opposing groups of muscles. Tremor is extremely variable in type and severity. Intention tremor is a coarse tremor that disappears when the animal is at rest. Intention tremor is most obvious in the head, where it appears as vibration of the head in a dorsoventral or craniocaudal direction. Having the patient stretch out his neck to accept a piece of food exacerbates intention tremor.

- Other types of tremors are variable in type and severity. They may affect a single limb or the entire body and have a legion of different causes (see Table 6).

CLINICAL NEUROANATOMY

- Abnormalities of gait and movement occur with lesions throughout the nervous system, including the brain stem, cerebellum, spinal cord, peripheral nerves, neuromuscular junction, and musculature.

- Common types of abnormalities and the possible locations for the lesions causing these abnormalities are listed in Table 6.

- Further details of the neuroanatomical basis of gait and gait abnormalities are presented in the discussion of proprioception and the postural reactions (see Chapter 7).

TABLE 6

Location of Lesions Causing Gait and Movement Disorders

Clinical Sign	Location of Lesions	Distinguishing Features
Quadriparesis/ quadriplegia and ataxia of all four limbs	Midbrain	Decreased consciousness, decerebrate posture, and other signs of midbrain disease
	Medulla oblongata	Vestibular or cranial nerve involement
	Cervical spinal cord C_1-C_5	Normal brain; normal to increased reflexes in all limbs
	Cervical spinal cord C_6-T_2	Normal brain; decreased reflexes in forelimbs, increased reflexes in hind limbs
	Diffuse neuropathy, myopathy, or neuromuscular junction disease	Normal brain; decreased reflexes in all limbs (neuropathy) or normal reflexes in all limbs (myopathy); variable reflexes in neuromuscular junction disease; variable muscle atrophy
Hemiparesis and ataxia	Contralateral midbrain, ipsilateral medulla oblongata, ipsilateral spinal cord C_1-C_5 or C_6-T_2	As above for each site
Paraparesis/ paraplegia and ataxia	Spinal cord T_3-L_3	Normal to increased reflexes in hind limbs; +/- Schiff-Sherrington syndrome
	Spinal cord L_4-S_2	Decreased reflexes in hind limbs; Schiff-Sherrington syndrome unusual

TABLE 6 (continued)

Localization of Lesions Causing Gait and Movement Disorders

Clinical Sign	Localization of Lesions	Distinguishing Features
Dysmetria, hypermetria	Cerebellum	Other signs of cerebellar disease, such as intention tremor and loss of menace reflex with normal vision
	Spinal cord	Involvement of spino-cerebellar tracts in spinal cord can cause mild to moderate hypermetria without other signs of cerebellar dysfunction
Tremor	Cerebellum	Intention tremor disappears at rest and worsens with movement
	Diffuse brain; peripheral nerve lesions	A wide variety of clinical signs are possible; may be difficult to localize lesion

CLINICAL TIPS

- The neurological control of gait is best evaluated when the patient is moved at a brisk walk, rather than a trot.

7

Proprioception and the Postural Reactions

Proprioception is a term that describes the sense of position in space, independent of visual information. Proprioception in humans is the sense that permits a person to touch his or her nose with a fingertip even when the eyes are closed. Proprioception is both conscious (i.e., the incoming sensory information on body position reaches the cerebral cortex) and unconscious, primarily involving vestibular and cerebellar centers in the brain stem.

The postural reactions tested during the neurological examination help to determine the integrity of the sensory and motor pathways involved in gait. Virtually the entire nervous system, from receptors in the limbs to the cerebral cortex and back to the muscles, is involved when the postural reactions are tested. Abnormality anywhere in the ascending or descending components of the pathways tested will produce the same clinical signs.

All the postural reaction tests involve essentially the same pathways. In the course of a typical neurological examination, it is necessary only to examine gait, then test proprioception and hopping in each limb. Other postural reactions are useful, though, in some circumstances.

FORELIMB PROPRIOCEPTION

NEUROLOGICAL EXAMINATION

- The animal should be standing. Place one hand under the chest, either between or just behind the forelimbs. If the animal can support his own weight, the hand is there just to steady him and prevent him from tipping to one side when the foot is lifted. If the animal is weak or unable to stand, then the examiner must support him in an upright position.

- In animals that are unable to stand, a second person may be needed to support the animal's hind end.

- Lift one foot and turn it over, so that the dorsum of the paw is on the floor or table.

- Alternatively, have the animal stand with one front foot on a piece of paper. Pull the paper laterally quite slowly.

HIND LIMB PROPRIOCEPTION

NEUROLOGICAL EXAMINATION

- The animal should be standing. Stand behind the animal, reach between his back legs, and place a hand just under the pubis. The edge of the hand, not the palm, should be against the pubis.

- Avoid curling the fingers of the supporting hand around the front of the patient's thigh or placing the hand around the abdomen immediately in front of the thigh. It is the author's experience that this frequently causes a slow response, even in normal animals.

- With small dogs and cats, a single finger will suffice to provide support.

- With heavy dogs, the elbow of the supporting hand can be rested on the examiner's knee to help support the patient's weight.

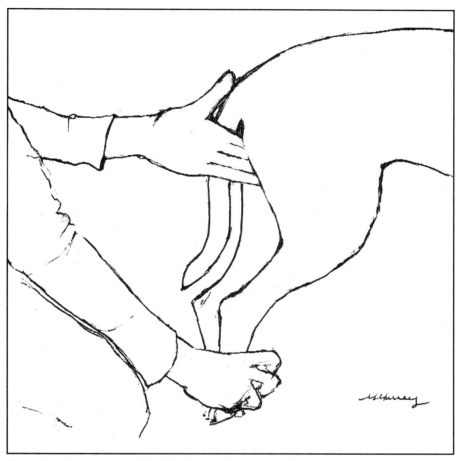

Figure 10. Examination, Hind Limb Proprioception. *Lift one foot and turn it over, so that the dorsum of the paw is on the floor or table.*

- The hand is in place to provide a little support and steadiness for animals with good strength or a lot of support for weak animals. For very weak animals, a second person may be needed to support the forelimbs.

- Lift one foot and turn it over, so that the dorsum of the paw is on the floor or table (Figure 10).

- As with the forelimb, an alternative method for testing proprioception is to place the animal's foot on a piece of paper laid on the floor or table and slowly pull the paper laterally.

NORMAL FINDINGS

- Immediately after the examiner releases the foot that has been turned over, the patient should lift it and replace it into a normal, pad-down position.

- It is common for animals with normal proprioception to strongly resist having the foot placed with the dorsum of the paw on the table or floor. Sometimes the examiner cannot place the animal's foot in the dorsum-down position.

- Resistance to having the foot placed in an abnormal position is usually very strong in cats.

- When the animal's foot is placed on a piece of paper, and the paper is pulled laterally, the normal response is for the animal to lift the foot almost as soon as the foot is lateral to the lateral margins of the trunk. He will then replace the foot closer to the midline.

ABNORMAL FINDINGS

- The patient leaves the foot in an abnormal position, with the dorsum of the paw against the table or floor, or he replaces it into a pad-down position more slowly than normal.

- The animal allows the limb to be drawn laterally and does not replace it closer to the midline, or he does so only after the limb has been pulled a long way to one side.

FORELIMB HOPPING

NEUROLOGICAL EXAMINATION

- Stand to the left side of the patient, level with his hip. Reach over his back and place your right arm and hand under his abdomen.

- Place your left hand on the cranial aspect of the patient's upper arm, just above the elbow.

- Flex the patient's elbow so his forelimb is lifted a few inches above the floor. Lift the hind limbs a few inches off the floor (Figure 11).

- Force the patient to hop toward the right on the right fore-limb by turning your body clockwise (Figure 12). Do not walk with the patient, but stand in one place and turn your body in a circle.

- Have the patient hop six steps or more, until you are comfortable that you can assess the strength and speed of his hopping.

- Repeat the process to test the left forelimb.

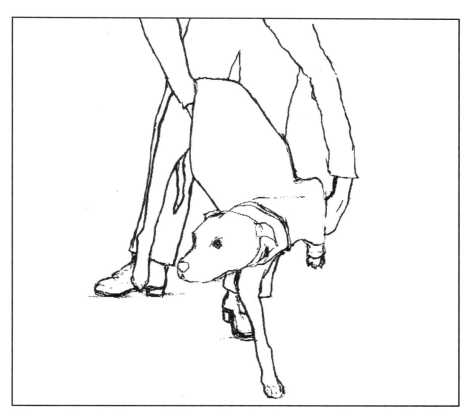

Figure 11. Examination, Forelimb Hopping. *Flex the patient's elbow so his forelimb is lifted a few inches above the floor.*

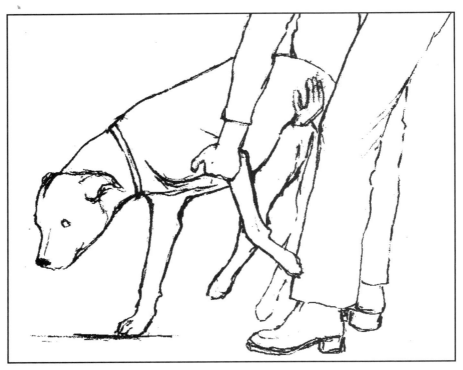

Figure 12. Examination, Forelimb Hopping. *Force the patient to hop toward the right on the right forelimb by turning your body clockwise.*

HIND LIMB HOPPING

NEUROLOGICAL EXAMINATION

- Stand at the left side of the patient, facing his hind limbs. Reach across his back just behind the forelimbs and under the chest or in front of the left shoulder and between his forelimbs, placing your hand under the sternum (Figure 13). Place your right hand on the back of his thigh, just above the stifle joint.

- Flex the hind limb at the stifle and hip so that the foot clears the floor by a couple of inches (Figure 14). Lift the forelimbs a few inches off the ground.

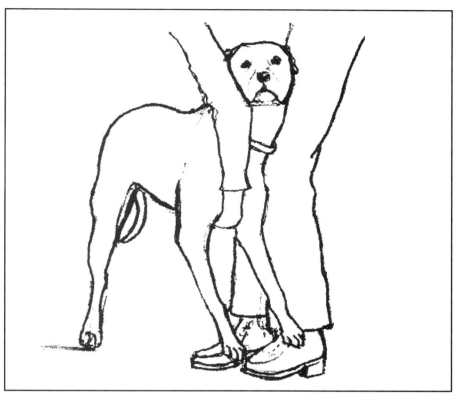

Figure 13. Examination, Hind Limb Hopping. *Place one hand under the chest to steady the animal.*

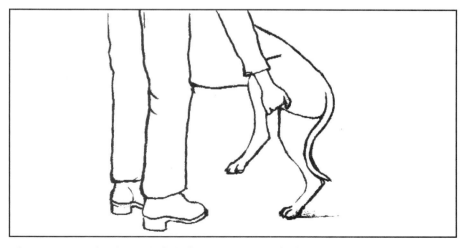

Figure 14. Examination, Hind Limb Hopping. *Flex the hind limb at the stifle and hip so that the foot clears the floor by a couple of inches.*

- Force the patient to hop toward the left on the right hind limb by turning your body counterclockwise. Do not walk with the patient, but stand in one place and turn your body in a circle.

- Have the patient hop at least six steps or more, until you are comfortable that you can assess the strength and speed of his hopping.

- Repeat the process to test the left hind limb.

NORMAL FINDINGS

- The patient will briskly hop on the limb being tested, supporting most of his weight on that limb.

ABNORMAL FINDINGS

- The patient may be unable to support weight on the limb being tested, may buckle or knuckle the foot, may not attempt to hop, or may hop very slowly.

CLINICAL TIPS

- Ensure that you test hopping on a non-slip surface with good traction. A rubber mat is ideal. Otherwise, concrete, tarmac, or grass may provide a better surface than most examination-room floors.

- Cats and small dogs can be tested on the examination table. Again, a rubber mat will provide good traction. Alternatively, kneel on the floor to test smaller patients.

- Force the animal to bear much of his weight on the limb being tested. If the response is poor, try having him bear more weight on the limb, unless it is obvious that he is too weak to do so.

- Move the animal quite briskly in a circle around you. If he seems reluctant to cooperate, moving him a little faster may help.

- Always have the patient hop toward the lateral aspect of the limb (i.e., to the right, or clockwise, for the right forelimb and left hind limb; and to the left, or counterclockwise, for the left forelimb and right hind limb). It is much more difficult for animals to hop toward the medial aspect of the limbs and, therefore, more difficult for the clinician to assess normal versus abnormal responses.

- If you are dealing with a large or heavy patient, have an assistant lift one end of the patient while you lift the other. If no assistant is available, try using the hemiwalking and/or wheelbarrowing tests instead of the hopping test. It is easier to perform the hopping test in animals that are long in body (e.g., greyhounds) when two people can help.

HEMIWALKING

NEUROLOGICAL EXAMINATION

- Stand facing the right flank of the patient.

- Place your right hand on his right forelimb just above the elbow, as you did when testing hopping.

- Place your left hand on the caudal aspect of his right thigh, just above the stifle joint, also as you did for hopping.

- Flex the forelimb slightly at the elbow and shoulder and the hind limb at the stifle and hip, so that both limbs are a few inches off the ground (Figure 15).

- Push the patient toward his left (i.e., away from you) and move with him as he moves away from you.

NORMAL FINDINGS

- The animal should be able to take coordinated steps away from you without falling.

ABNORMAL FINDINGS

- The animal may be weak or ataxic and could fall as you push him away from you.

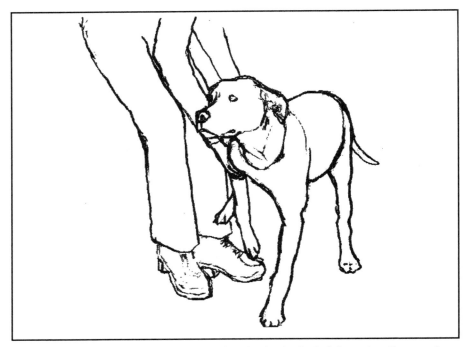

Figure 15. Examination, Hemiwalking. *Flex the forelimb slightly at the elbow and shoulder and the hind limb at the stifle and hip.*

CLINICAL TIPS

- Ensure that you keep your hands under the patient's shoulder and hip, and avoid pulling his limbs laterally. Doing so will possibly tip him over and may cause even a normal animal to fall.

- If you are concerned that the patient may fall, have an assistant stand on the patient's opposite side, ready to catch him should he start to fall.

- If gait, proprioception, and hopping are normal, it is not necessary to test hemiwalking.

- Hemiwalking is a good test for detecting subtle differences between one side of the body and the other.

- Hemiwalking is useful when the patient is too large for you to test hopping single-handedly.

WHEELBARROWING

NEUROLOGICAL EXAMINATION

- Stand behind the patient and place your hands around his caudal abdomen.

- Lift his hind limbs a few inches above the floor and push him forward, so he walks on his forelimbs only (Figure 16).

- Next, stand facing the patient and place your hands around his thorax, supporting him under the sternum.

- Lift his forelimbs a few inches above the floor and walk backward, causing him to walk forward on his hind limbs only.

NORMAL FINDINGS

- The patient walks forward on his forelimbs alone and on his hind limbs alone in a normal, coordinated fashion.

ABNORMAL FNDINGS

- He shows evidence of ataxia, weakness, incoordination, or other gait abnormalities.

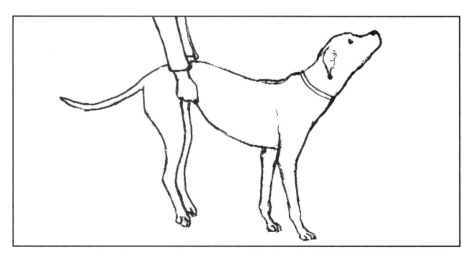

Figure 16. Examination, Wheelbarrowing. *Lift his hind limbs a few inches above the floor and push him forward.*

CLINICAL TIPS

- Do not raise the limbs more than a few inches off the floor. An exaggerated, hyperextended body posture makes walking on two limbs difficult even for normal animals.

- Always have the patient walk forward, either on both forelimbs or on both hind limbs. Walking backward is more difficult and results in a stiff, stilted gait. This may make it difficult to distinguish normal from mildly abnormal animals.

- Wheelbarrowing is useful for comparing forelimb gait and hind limb gait. It also can be used when you are examining a large or heavy patient and have no assistant to help you test hopping.

PLACING REACTIONS

NEUROLOGICAL EXAMINATION

- In large dogs, visual placing can be tested by having the patient climb and descend stairs.

- If necessary, tactile placing can be tested by blindfolding the patient before he climbs or descends the stairs.

- For small dogs and cats, lift the animal up and hold him so that one forelimb is free. With the patient facing the examination table, bring his body toward the edge of the table. Test both forelimbs in turn.

- Repeat the test while either covering the patient's eyes (an assistant can help with this) or holding his head up so he can't see the table. Bring the patient forward until his foot just touches the edge of the table.

- Now, turn his body so that his side faces the table. The hind limb closest to the table should be free. Bring the dog toward the table until the hind foot closest to the table touches the edge of the table.

NORMAL FINDINGS

- Animals ascend and descend stairs in a coordinated fashion.

- When the patient can see the table and once he is close to the table, he should reach out with his foot and place it on the table.

- When his eyes are covered or his head is held up so he cannot see the table, he should reach out and place his foot on the table immediately after the foot touches the edge of the table.

- When the hind limbs are being tested, the patient should reach out and place his foot on the table immediately after the foot touches the edge of the table.

ABNORMAL FINDINGS

- The patient shows evidence of weakness, ataxia, or other gait abnormalities when ascending or descending stairs.

- He does not place his foot on the table when placing is tested as described above.

CLINICAL TIPS

- Ensure that the patient is used to stairs. Occasionally, animals are presented that have never climbed stairs. They may be reluctant to do so and appear stiff or weak when they first attempt it.

- A "bunny-hopping" hind limb gait may be normal in small dogs when they ascend stairs rapidly. Have the owner move them more slowly up the stairs. Short-legged breeds, like Welsh corgis, may still bunny-hop. Bunny-hopping is not usual in larger dogs. If this gait persists despite a slower pace, it suggests a lesion in the sensory or motor pathway for control of gait (see the following discussion on "Clinical Neuroanatomy of Gait"). Bunny-hopping when walking on a level surface is abnormal in all animals.

- Small dogs and cats, particularly those that are held much of the time, may be unwilling to attempt placing, even when they are otherwise normal.

- If the patient does not place, try holding him a little further away from you, so that he feels less secure.

- Most animals resent having their eyes covered. Holding the head up so that the patient cannot see the table is often a better alternative when testing placing.

- If you find that the patient is anticipating the table when you are testing tactile placing, try moving to another side of the table or discontinue the test and return to it later.

CLINICAL NEUROANATOMY OF GAIT, PROPRIOCEPTION, AND THE POSTURAL REACTIONS

- The mechanisms underlying the control of gait and the postural reactions are complex and involve almost all parts of the nervous system. A detailed description is beyond the scope of this text, and the reader is referred to the sources listed in Appendix 3. The following is a brief overview.

- The major motor centers in the brain lie in the brain stem (i.e., midbrain, pons, and medulla). Voluntary movement may be initiated within the brain stem or in the motor area in the frontal lobe of the cerebral cortex. Input from the basal nuclei (i.e., basal ganglia) vestibular system and cerebellum also influences activity in the brain-stem motor centers. There are many interconnections between all these central components of the motor systems. Axons from neurons whose cell bodies lie in the brain-stem motor centers descend the spinal cord in several tracts (i.e., rubrospinal, reticulospinal, tectospinal, vestibulospinal), which lie predominantly in the lateral and ventral funiculi of the spinal cord. These descending neurons (i.e., upper-motor neurons) synapse on lower-motor neurons in the spinal cord ventral-horn gray matter. The axons of the lower-motor neurons emerge from the spinal cord and form the peripheral nerves to the limbs. Pathways that descend directly from the cerebral motor cortex to the lower-motor neurons (i.e., corticospinal pathways) are of relatively little importance in quadrupeds. The motor pathways cross the midline in the caudal midbrain and rostral medulla oblongata, so lesions in the brain rostral to this point cause contralateral ataxia and paresis, whereas lesions caudal to this point cause ipsilateral ataxia and paresis. Vestibular and cerebellar control of gait is ipsilateral.

- Lesions in the sensory pathways that are involved in the control of gait also cause abnormalities of gait and the postural reactions. The major sensory pathways for position sense (i.e., proprioception) lie in the dorsal and dorsolateral areas of the spinal cord. Information for proprioceptors in the joints, muscles, and skin is conveyed to the cerebral cortex via the gracile and cuneate fascicles in the dorsal funiculus of the spinal cord. This system is also called the medial lemniscal system. This information reaches the cerebral cortex as conscious proprioception, which is tested by means of turning over the foot (as previously described) as well as by means of the postural reactions. The medial lemniscal pathway crosses the midline in the rostral medulla oblongata, so information from one side of the body is perceived in the opposite cerebral hemisphere.

- Unconscious proprioception refers to information from the limbs that is conveyed cranially to the brain stem and the cerebellum via pathways in the lateral and dorsolateral aspects of the spinal cord (i.e., spinocerebellar and spinothalamic tracts). Ascending information conveyed to the cerebellum remains ipsilateral, whereas pathways ascending to the thalamus cross the midline in the rostral medulla oblongata.

- Both lesions in the ascending (i.e., sensory) and descending (i.e., motor) components, as well as those affecting lower-motor neurons or muscles directly, can cause abnormalities of gait and postural reactions. Proprioceptive deficits suggest abnormalities in the sensory pathways (mainly the medial lemniscal system), but weakness caused by motor system lesions may result in an animal that has normal proprioception but lacks the strength to replace the foot in a normal position when conscious proprioception is tested.

- It is difficult, if not impossible, to differentiate between lesions in the sensory and motor components of the CNS control of gait on the basis of the clinical neurological examination; it also is not considered necessary in most cases. Most lesions in the CNS, particularly within the spinal cord, involve both motor and sensory systems.

8

Myotactic Reflexes

The myotactic reflexes are elicited to help determine the longitudinal location of a lesion within the spinal cord or affecting the peripheral nerves.

PATELLAR REFLEX

NEUROLOGICAL EXAMINATION

- The patellar reflex is the most easily elicited of all the myotactic reflexes.

- The animal should be lying in lateral recumbency, and the reflex should be tested in the limb on the uppermost side.

- Flex the limb at the stifle joint to an angle of about sixty degrees.

- Support the limb being tested slightly above the opposite limb by placing your hand beneath the stifle, with your open palm supporting the medial aspect of the joint (Figure 17).

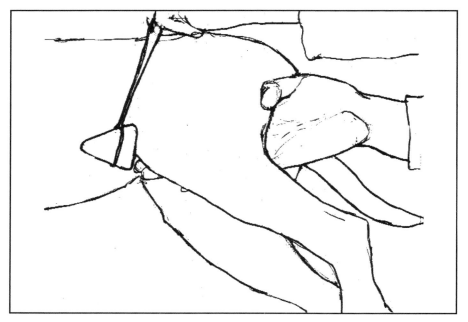

Figure 17. Examination of the Patellar Reflex. *Support the limb being tested slightly above the opposite limb by placing your hand beneath the stifle, with your open palm supporting the medial aspect of the joint.*

- Hold the percussion hammer perpendicular to the patellar tendon. The handle of the hammer should be almost vertical.

- Percuss the tendon sharply at its midpoint using the flat edge of the hammer.

NORMAL FINDINGS

- The normal response is for the quadriceps femoris muscle to contract, causing the limb distal to the stifle joint to swing forward.

ABNORMAL FINDINGS

- When upper-motor neuron disease is present (i.e., lesions in the spinal cord cranial to L_4 or lesions in the brain), the reflex movement is exaggerated and a brisk response may be elicited by a minimal stimulus.

- With severe upper-motor neuron disease, a clonic response may occur. In clonus, the reflex response is repeated several times in quick succession. The limb seems to "oscillate" or "reverberate."

- When lower-motor neuron disease is present (i.e., lesions in spinal cord segments L_4-L_6; in spinal nerve roots or spinal nerves originating from these cord segments; or in the femoral nerve, neuromuscular junctions, or quadriceps femoris muscle), the reflex movement is weak or may be absent.

- A "pseudohyperreflexia" may occur when lower-motor neuron lesions are present, affecting the sciatic nerve. Such lesions cause weakness in the caudal thigh muscles, which normally oppose the action of the quadriceps femoris muscle (e.g., lesions in spinal-cord segments L_6-S_1; in spinal nerve roots or spinal nerves originating from these cord segments; or in the sciatic nerve, neuromuscular junctions, or caudal thigh group of muscles). When the patellar reflex is elicited in these circumstances, the forward movement of the lower limb produced by contraction of the quadriceps is not opposed by the normal muscle tone of the caudal thigh muscles, permitting the limb to jerk forward more than normal. This situation is differentiated from that caused by true upper-motor neuron lesions by the presence of other signs of lesions affecting spinal-cord segments L_4-L_6 or in the sciatic nerve (e.g., decreased withdrawal [i.e., flexion] reflex in the affected limb, decreased gastrocnemius and cranial tibial muscle reflexes, and neurogenic atrophy of muscles innervated by the sciatic nerve).

CLINICAL TIPS

- Some animals are very resistant to being held in lateral recumbency. The usual reason for this resistance is that animals perceive this as a submissive posture.

- Resistance can usually be overcome by using reassuring tones when speaking to the animal and using gentle but firm handling. Putting a hand across the bridge of the nose may help; this increases the handler's dominance and may cause the animal to "give in." Placing a hand or fore-arm across the neck when the animal is recumbent, or applying a muzzle to animals that threaten to bite, may help. Shouting or vigorous physical struggles are not helpful.

- Animals often flex the hind limbs when recumbent, mak-ing examination of the patellar reflex difficult. Hold the flexed limb just below the hock joint and gently flex and extend the limb a few times; this may help the animal to relax. If the animal flexes the limb when you support it with your hand under the stifle, try testing the reflex without supporting the limb. If this does not help, hold the limb below the hock and extend it until the angle at the stifle is about sixty degrees; then test the patellar reflex.

- Scratching the animal's belly to encourage the animal to relax often causes him to increase the flexion of the limb and to abduct the limb to "encourage" the belly rub, thus defeating the handler's objective!

- On rare occasions, animals will not relax sufficiently for the reflex to be tested. In such cases, other signs, such as the mass and tone of the quadriceps femoris muscle, must be used to help differentiate between upper- and lower-motor neuron disease.

- Animals that are tense and increase their muscle tone suffi-ciently to prevent myotactic reflexes from being tested are like-ly to have normal to increased muscle tone, consistent with a normal nervous system or the presence of upper-motor neu-ron disease, rather than lower-motor neuron disease.

- In cats and small dogs, it may be helpful to use a smaller instrument, such as the handle of a hemostat, rather than a percussion hammer. Alternatively, place a fingertip over the patellar tendon and percuss the back of the finger, which transfers the force directly to the tendon.

CRANIAL TIBIAL REFLEX

NEUROLOGICAL EXAMINATION

- Hold the hind limb at the hock, with the limb in a relaxed position.

- Strike the middle of the cranial tibial muscle sharply, using the pointed end of the percussion hammer (Figure 18).

NORMAL FINDINGS

- The cranial tibial muscle contracts, flexing the hock.

ABNORMAL FINDINGS

- The reflex is increased, clonic, or decreased to absent.

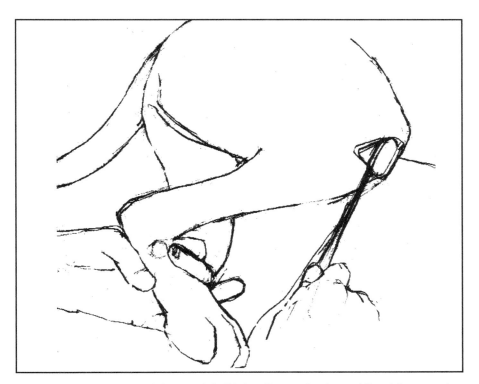

Figure 18. Examination of the Cranial Tibial Reflex. *Strike the middle of the cranial tibial muscle sharply, using the pointed end of the percussion hammer.*

CLINICAL TIPS

- To facilitate the reflex, stretch the cranial tibial muscle slightly by holding the limb below the hock, extending the stifle slightly, and then flexing the hock slightly. Now percuss the muscle. Since you are holding the leg below the hock and causing the position of the hock to be flexed, the reflex contraction will be perceived as a slight flexion of the stifle.

GASTROCNEMIUS REFLEX

NEUROLOGICAL EXAMINATION

- Hold the hind limb below the hock, with the hock moderately flexed and the stifle slightly extended.

- Using the flat end of the percussion hammer, strike the gastrocnemius tendon (Achilles tendon) just above its attachment to the calcaneus, or strike the middle of the gastrocnemius muscle sharply, using the pointed end of the percussion hammer (Figure 19).

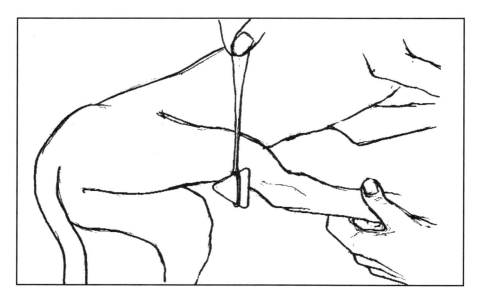

Figure 19. Examination of the Gastrocnemius Reflex. Using the flat end of the percussion hammer, strike the gastrocnemius tendon.

NORMAL FINDINGS

- The gastrocnemius muscle contracts, extending the hock.

ABNORMAL FINDINGS

- The reflex is increased, clonic, or decreased to absent.

CLINICAL TIPS

- Holding the hock in moderate flexion facilitates the reflex.

SCIATIC REFLEX

NEUROLOGICAL EXAMINATION

- The leg being tested should be in a relaxed position. Place the tip of a finger over the sciatic notch, between the greater trochanter of the femur and the ischiatic tuberosity. Strike the back of the finger sharply with the pointed end of the percussion hammer.

NORMAL FINDINGS

- The limb flexes at both stifle and hock.

ABNORMAL FINDINGS

- Absence of limb movement indicates lower-motor neuron disease.

CLINICAL TIPS

- This is not a true reflex, but rather the sciatic nerve is stimulated directly as it runs through the sciatic notch. This response can be elicited for several minutes postmortem, so its value is debatable! It is true to say, however, that the response is often absent in severe lower-motor neuron disease affecting the sciatic nerve or its origins in the spinal cord. In this instance, the findings do have some clinical significance.

TRICEPS REFLEX

NEUROLOGICAL EXAMINATION

- Hold the forelimb with the elbow flexed at about ninety degrees. Pull the limb forward (toward the animal's nose) slightly, until you feel moderate resistance.

- Percuss the triceps tendon just above its insertion at the olecranon (Figure 20).

NORMAL FINDINGS

- The elbow is retracted and extended.

- The contraction of the triceps muscle itself may be visible in short-coated animals.

ABNORMAL FINDINGS

- The reflex response may be decreased to absent or increased to clonic.

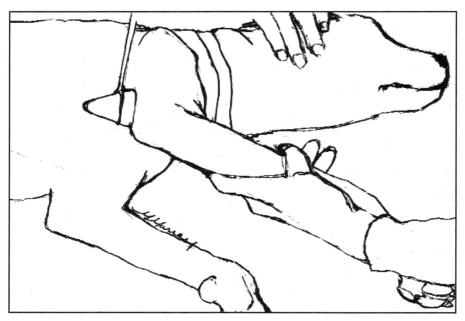

Figure 20. Examination of the Triceps Reflex. *Percuss the triceps tendon just above its insertion at the olecranon.*

CLINICAL TIPS

- Percussing slightly toward the medial aspect of the tendon often facilitates the reflex.

- For small dogs and cats, it may be helpful to use an instrument smaller than a percussion hammer, such as the handle of a hemostat.

- For small dogs and cats, or for dogs that have a lot of loose skin on the caudal aspect of the elbow, place a fingertip over the triceps tendon and percuss the back of the finger using the pointed end of the reflex hammer. This transfers the force from the hammer to the tendon.

BICEPS REFLEX

NEUROLOGICAL EXAMINATION

- Abduct the uppermost limb slightly and hold it in relaxed extension.

- Curl the index finger of your nondominant hand around the cranial aspect of the elbow to palpate the biceps tendon, which lies on the anteromedial aspect of the elbow.

- Percuss the finger lying on the biceps tendon, using the pointed end of the reflex hammer (Figure 21).

- An alternative method is as follows. Retract the uppermost limb, exposing the medial aspect of the elbow of the limb closest to the ground.

- Place the index finger of your nondominant hand on the biceps tendon of the lower limb.

- Percuss the finger lying on the biceps tendon, using the pointed end of the reflex hammer.

NORMAL FINDINGS

- The elbow flexes slightly, and the contraction of the biceps muscle (which lies on the anteromedial aspect of the limb, overlying the humerus) may be visible in short-coated breeds.

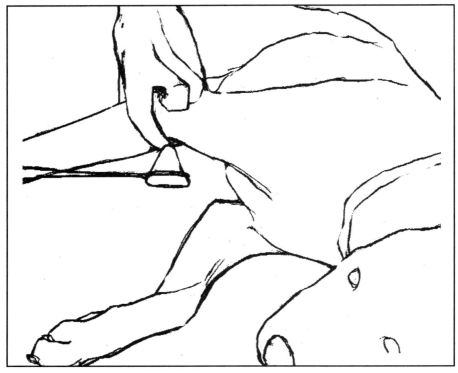

Figure 21. Examination of the Biceps Reflex. *Percuss the finger lying on the biceps tendon.*

ABNORMAL FINDINGS

- The reflex response may be decreased to absent or increased to clonic.

CLINICAL TIPS

- The biceps reflex is probably the most difficult myotactic reflex to elicit. If muscle mass, proprioception, hopping, and gait are normal, it is unlikely that there is a lesion affecting the biceps muscle or its innervation, even in animals where this reflex cannot be elicited.

- When testing the reflex in the uppermost part of the limb, it is helpful to have an assistant support the lower part of the limb by placing a hand below the carpus.

EXTENSOR CARPI REFLEX

NEUROLOGICAL EXAMINATION

- Hold the uppermost limb by supporting it in the middle of the radius, having both the elbow and carpus in a relaxed but flexed position.

- Percuss the extensor carpi muscle directly, using the pointed end of the percussion hammer, about one to three inches distal to the elbow (depending on the size of the patient) (Figure 22). The muscle lies slightly lateral to the dorsal aspect of the limb.

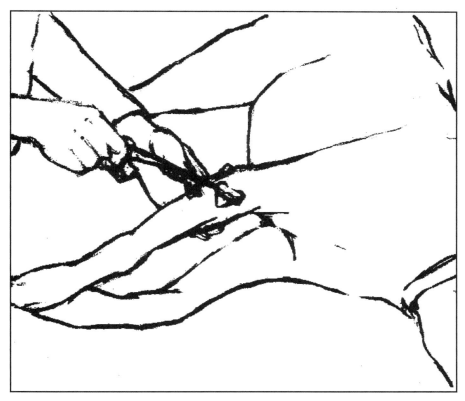

Figure 22. Examination of the Extensor Carpi Reflex. *Percuss the extensor carpi muscle directly, using the pointed end of the percussion hammer, about one to three inches distal to the elbow.*

NORMAL FINDINGS

- The carpus extends.

ABNORMAL FINDINGS

- The reflex response may be decreased to absent or increased to clonic.

CLINICAL TIPS

- In this author's experience, the extensor carpi reflex may be present even in animals known to have lesions of the radial nerve (e.g., brachial plexus avulsion). This suggests that the response is largely a mechanical one, caused by physical deformation of the muscle when it is percussed. The value of this reflex in assessing neurological function, therefore, is dubious.

ESSENTIAL NEUROANATOMY OF THE MYOTACTIC REFLEXES

The neuroanatomic principles underlying the myotactic reflexes are similar in all cases and are outlined below.

- The tendon of the muscle is stretched by tapping it with a reflex hammer. This action stretches the entire muscle, including the many muscle spindles that are located in each myofiber.

- Stretching the muscle spindles stimulates the stretch receptors within each spindle, which produces an action potential in the sensory nerve that innervates the spindles.

- The action potential travels centrally within the sensory neurons, which enter the spinal cord via the dorsal roots of spinal cord segments.

- One branch of the sensory neuron terminates by synapsing on a motor neuron in the ventral horn gray matter of the same spinal cord segment.

	TABLE 7	
	Neuroanatomy of the Myotactic Reflexes	
Reflex	**Muscle**	**Peripheral Nerve and Spinal Origin Muscle**
Biceps	Biceps brachii	Musculocutaneous; C_6-C_8
Extensor carpi	Extensor carpi radialis	Radial; C_7-T_2
Triceps	Triceps brachii	Radial; C_7-T_2
Patellar	Quadriceps femoris	Femoral; L_4-L_6
Gastrocnemius	Gastrocnemius	Sciatic; L_6-S_2
Cranial tibial	Cranial tibial	Sciatic; L_6-S_2
Sciatic	All hind-limb muscles with sciatic innervation	Sciatic; L_6-S_2

- The axon of the motor neuron exits the spinal cord in the ventral root of that same spinal cord segment, descends the hind limb within the peripheral nerve, and terminates at neuromuscular junctions within the muscle.

- Neuromuscular transmission at the junction results in the generation of an action potential within the myofibers inner-vated by that axon, causing contraction of the myofiber. Contraction of numerous myofibers results in contraction of the entire muscle, which is the reflex response.

- Lesions at the level of the reflex arc (either in the muscle, the peripheral nerve, the neuromuscular junctions, or the local spinal cord segments) cause decreased to absent reflex strength. Lesions rostral to the level of the reflex arc cause no change in the reflex or increased strength of the reflex. The detailed mechanisms by which changes in reflexes occur in nervous system disease are beyond the scope of this text. The neuroanatomy of the major myotactic reflexes is shown in Table 7.

9

Other Reflexes

Several reflexes in addition to the myotactic reflexes are helpful in localizing neurological lesions. The most dependable and commonly used of these reflexes are described here.

PANNICULUS REFLEX

NEUROLOGICAL EXAMINATION

- Using mosquito forceps, pinch the skin on either side of the body at the level of the cranial edge of the wings of the ilium (Figure 23). If no response is elicited after three or four attempts in several areas, move the stimulus cranially by one to three inches until a response is elicited or until you reach the level of the caudal part of the scapulae. Remember that this stimulus is painful, and the animal may object if you repeat the test too many times!

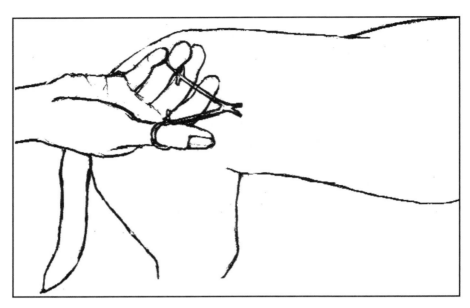

Figure 23. Examination of the Panniculus Reflex. Using mosquito forceps, pinch the skin on either side of the body at the level of the cranial edge of the wings of the ilium.

NORMAL FINDINGS

- A wrinkling of the skin over the dorsum should occur in response to the skin pinch, as a result of contraction of the cutaneous trunci muscle. This response should be elicited when the skin is pinched at or just cranial to the cranial edge of the ilium.

ABNORMAL FINDINGS

- The reflex may be absent on one or both sides at the level of the cranial ilium, but it may be elicited when the skin is pinched further rostrally. The level at which the reflex is elicited should be noted. The reflex may be completely absent on one side of the body or, rarely, on both sides.

CLINICAL NEUROANATOMY

- Sensory information from the skin of the trunk is conveyed to the spinal cord along cutaneous branches of the segmental spinal nerves. The neurons of the sensory pathway travel cranially in the spinal cord until they synapse bilaterally on the lower motor neurons of the lateral thoracic nerves in spinal cord segments C_8-T_1. Activation of these motor neurons results in the skin twitch.

- The skin of the trunk is innervated by segmental spinal nerves. The nerves emerge from the spinal canal and run slightly caudal before supplying sensory innervation to the skin. The further caudal along the body wall, the further caudal the nerves travel before innervating the skin. Thus, the skin at the level of the T_1 vertebral body is innervated by segmental spinal nerves originating from the T_1 spinal cord segment, whereas the skin at the level of L_6 is innervated by spinal nerves originating in the L_2 spinal cord segment.

- Knowledge of this pattern of innervation of the trunk can be used to facilitate localization of spinal cord lesions. When the panniculus reflex is absent caudal to a certain point on the trunk, the lesion in the spinal cord is located immediately rostral to the site of origin of the spinal nerves innervating that region of the trunk. For example, a lesion causing loss of the panniculus caudal to the thoracolumbar junction is located in the vicinity of the T_{10} spinal cord segment.

- Lesions involving the C_8 and T_1 spinal cord segments and the motor neurons of the lateral thoracic nerve may cause complete absence of the reflex on the ipsilateral side of the body, or even bilaterally, if the lesion is severe.

CLINICAL TIPS

- In heavy-coated breeds, ensure that the pinch stimulus is being applied to the skin.

- The reflex may be absent in a small number of normal animals.

- Obese animals, or those with generalized neuropathies or myopathies (such as those that may result from hyperadrenocorticism or hypothyroidism) sometimes lack the panniculus reflex while not having other evidence of spinal cord disease.

THE PERINEAL REFLEX AND TAIL TONE

NEUROLOGICAL EXAMINATION

- Handle the tail to evaluate its muscular strength. Touch the mucocutaneous junction at the anus with the tip of a closed hemostat (Figure 24).

NORMAL FINDINGS

- The tail should have normal tone and movement, consistent with the general size and strength of the patient.

- When the perianal area is touched, the anus contracts.

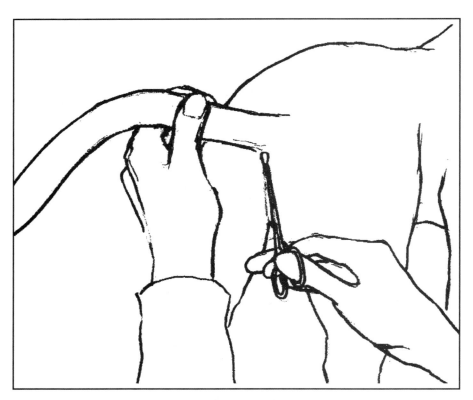

Figure 24. Examination of the Perineal Reflex and Tail Tone. Handle the tail to evaluate its muscular strength. Touch the mucocutaneous junction at the anus with the tip of a closed hemostat.

ABNORMAL FNDINGS

- Decreased to absent tail tone and movement. Decreased to absent response when the perianal area is touched.

CLINICAL NEUROANATOMY

- The tail is innervated by the coccygeal nerves, arising from the terminal portion of the spinal cord. The anal area is innervated by the pudendal nerve, which originates from the S_1-S_3 spinal cord segments. Loss of tail or anal tone results from lesions in the terminal portion of the spinal cord or of the nerves to these structures, which travel within the spinal canal as the cauda equina. The cauda equina originates at the termination of the spinal cord, usually within the L_5 vertebra, through the L_6 and L_7 vertebra and the sacrum. The coccygeal nerves continue into the tail.

CLINICAL TIPS

- Digital rectal examination is the most accurate method for determining anal strength.

- If feces are present in the rectum when a digital rectal examination is performed, the anal tone may be decreased, even in normal animals. Once the animal eliminates the fecal material, the anal tone will return to normal in normal animals.

FLEXOR (WITHDRAWAL) REFLEXES AND PERCEPTION OF PAIN

NEUROLOGICAL EXAMINATION

- When the patient is in lateral recumbency, apply an adverse stimulus (such as a pinch of the skin between the toes) to each foot in turn (Figure 25).

NORMAL FINDINGS

- The animal will flex (i.e., withdraw) the limb being tested and may demonstrate conscious recognition of the stimulus

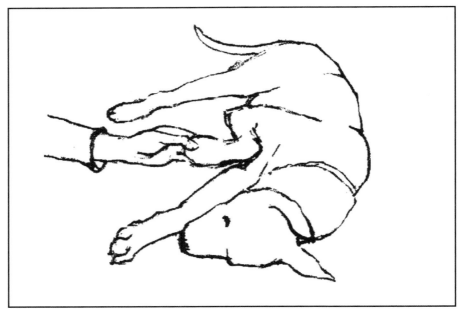

Figure 25. Examination of the Flexor Reflexes. *When the patient is in lateral recumbency, apply an adverse stimulus (such as a pinch of the skin between the toes) to each foot in turn.*

by turning the head, crying, or growling. The withdrawal should be strong (varying with the size of the patient) and all joints of the limb should be flexed.

ABNORMAL FINDINGS

- The animal does not withdraw the limb, withdrawal is weak, or the animal shows no conscious perception of the stimulus.

- Weak or absent withdrawal signifies dysfunction of the local motor or sensory components of the reflex: the peripheral nerve, the local spinal cord segments (C_6-T_2 for the forelimbs; L_4-S_2 for the hind limbs), or the limb musculature.

- Loss of conscious perception of pain results from interruption of the ascending pathway, either in the peripheral nerve, the spinal cord, or the brain. The spinal cord is the most common site of lesions that cause loss of pain perception in the limbs.

CLINICAL NEUROANATOMY

- The pathway for reflex withdrawal of the limb is a local one. Sensory information is transmitted in sensory neurons within the peripheral nerves innervating the area of skin being stimulated. This ascending information reaches local spinal cord segments and causes activation of spinal cord ventral horn cells, whose axons are motor-to-limb flexor muscles. Sensory information also ascends the spinal cord and reaches the cerebral cortex, resulting in conscious recognition of the stimulus.

- The sensation of pain is conveyed rostrally within the spinal cord in numerous pathways. These pathways are bilateral, and fibers cross the midline at numerous points. Both of these are features that tend to result in preservation of the sensory pathway for pain in the face of severe spinal cord disease. In very severe disease, however, even the sensation of deep pain, conveyed in small, unmyelinated nerve fibers, may be lost. Deep pain originates from the periosteum and is elicited by applying a strong pinch with a hemostat over a bone, such as a toe or the calcaneus.

- The initial stimulus for eliciting the flexor response is a pinch to the web of skin between two toes, applied with the fingers. If this does not result in flexion of the limb and conscious response to pain, the following stimuli can be applied in order of increasing severity: a hemostat pinch to the skin, a firm hemostat pinch to the base of a nail, and a firm hemostat pinch over the bone of a toe.

- Animals with severe lesions cranial to the origin of the peripheral nerves to a limb may have a loss of deep pain perception, with preservation of the local reflex of withdrawal of the limb in response to a skin pinch. The animal flexes the limb in response to the stimulus, but shows no signs that he perceives the pain. This usually signifies a poor prognosis. Withdrawal of the limb alone, without evidence of conscious awareness of pain, does not signify that pain perception is present.

THE CROSSED EXTENSOR REFLEX

NEUROLOGICAL EXAMINATION

- The crossed extensor reflex is a reflex extension of one limb when the opposite limb is flexed. When an animal is standing, it is a normal reflex and part of the subconscious mechanisms that control gait. This reflex is not specifically elicited during the neurological examination.

- When the flexor reflexes are tested, the limb being stimulated is flexed and the opposite limb extends.

NORMAL FINDINGS

- When an animal is in lateral recumbency, the crossed extensor reflex is inhibited.

ABNORMAL FINDINGS

- Severe, chronic spinal cord lesions (and occasionally brain lesions) that are rostral to the origins of the peripheral nerves to the limbs, may result in loss of descending inhibition of the crossed extensor reflex when the animal is recumbent.

- The presence of a crossed extensor reflex in a recumbent animal signifies a lesion ipsilateral to the limb that extends. The crossed extensor reflex does not necessarily signify a poor prognosis, as is often suggested.

CLINICAL TIPS

- Differentiate an abnormal crossed extensor reflex from voluntary efforts to escape the stimulus. Animals with a true abnormal crossed extensor reflex show a consistent and repeatable response, which occurs even when the animal is calm and relaxed. Animals trying to escape examination are usually anxious or excited, and their responses vary with repeated stimuli.

Neurological Examination Summary

OBSERVATION AT A DISTANCE

- Note the animal's behavior and level of alertness. Are these normal for this type and breed of animal under the conditions of the examination?

- Does vision appear normal? When moving around the room, does he avoid objects and appear to watch what is going on around him?

- Is there any abnormal posture, such as a head tilt?

- Observe the gait on a level surface and also on stairs, where appropriate.

- Check muscle mass. Is muscle mass adequate? Are both sides of the body symmetrical? Palpate the muscles and inspect them visually.

CRANIAL NERVE EXAMINATION

CN I – Olfactory

- Use a food substance to attract the animal's attention and see whether he will follow movement of the food with his nose. You may wish to blindfold the animal for this test.

CN II – Optic

- Test the menace reflex, covering the eye not being tested. Watch whether the animal will follow the path of a cotton ball dropped twelve to eighteen inches in front of him.

CN III – Oculomotor

- Observe the position of the globes within the orbits. Are they central in position?

- Test the oculocephalic reflexes by turning the head from side to side and up and down. Is the speed of the nystagmus normal and similar in all directions of head movement?

- Examine the size of the pupils. Are they appropriate for the light conditions and for the animal's level of excitement and anxiety? Are both pupils the same size?

- Test the pupillary light reflexes by shining a bright light in each eye in turn. Observe both the direct and indirect responses.

CN IV – Trochlear

- In the cat, is the orientation of the pupils normal?

- In the animal, lesions of the trochlear nerve are difficult to observe. Is the orientation of the retinal vasculature normal on fundic examination?

CN V – Trigeminal

- Stimulate both sides of the face using the tip of a closed hemostat. Does the animal respond by moving the muscles of the face (e.g., by blinking or wrinkling the lip)? Does he try to avoid the stimulus by pulling the head away, or otherwise demonstrate that he is conscious of the stimulus?

- Use a moistened cotton swab to touch the center of the cornea. Does the globe retract and does the animal try to avoid the stimulus?

- Examine the masseter and temporalis muscles both by observation and palpation. Are they a normal size for this type and size of animal? Are the muscles on both sides of the head symmetrical? Open the jaw. Is jaw strength normal?

CN VI – Abducent

- Are the positions of the globes within the orbits normal, or is there a medial strabismus?

- When the animal is looking around the room, does he have full range of movement of both eyes? Is the oculocephalic reflex normal in both eyes?

- When you touch the corneas while testing CN V function, do both globes retract?

CN VII – Facial

- Observe the face for symmetry. Is either the ear or lip drooping?

- When you test CN V function by touching the face, are the movements of the facial muscles normal?

CN VIII – Vestibulocochlear

- Does the animal have a head tilt or turn, or does he hold his head in a normal position?

- Was physiological nystagmus normal when you checked it earlier in the examination? Is spontaneous nystagmus present? This should be checked again later, with the animal lying on each side and on his back.

- Make a sound to one side or behind the animal, or have the owner call the animal's name. Does he alert and turn toward the sound?

CN IX and CN X – Glossopharyngeal and Vagus

- Test the gag response. Is the gag normal?

CN XII – Hypoglossal

- When testing the gag response, examine the size, shape, and movement of the tongue. Is the tongue normal in size and bilaterally symmetrical? Do tongue movements appear normal? Does the tongue deviate to either side?

CN XI – Accessory

- Palpate both sides of the neck and over the shoulder. Is the muscle mass normal in size and tone? Is the musculature symmetrical on both sides of the neck?

POSTURAL REACTIONS

Conscious Proprioception

- While supporting the animal appropriately, turn over each foot several times. Does the animal respond by briskly replacing each foot in a normal position?

- Conscious proprioception also can be tested using the "sliding paper" test.

Hopping

- Ensure adequate support for the animal and then have him hop on each leg in turn. Assess the strength and speed of his hopping response, as well as symmetry between right and left sides and between fore- and hind limbs.

Hemiwalking, Wheelbarrowing

- These tests are not compulsory but may be helpful when tests of gait, conscious proprioception, and hopping do not provide clear findings.

MYOTACTIC REFLEXES

- The animal should be placed in lateral recumbency. Check the eyes for nystagmus or strabismus. Now test the following reflexes:

Pelvic Limb

- Patellar reflex (femoral nerve; spinal cord segment L_4-L_6)

- Gastrocnemius reflex (sciatic/tibial nerve; spinal cord segments)

- Cranial tibial reflex

- Withdrawal response

- If the animal is severely paretic or paralyzed, test for superficial and deep pain perception.

Thoracic Limb

- Triceps reflex

- Biceps reflex

- Withdrawal response. Don't forget to watch for a crossed extensor response, which is abnormal in recumbent animals.

- If the animal is severely paretic or paralyzed, test for superficial and deep pain perception.

- Roll the animal onto his back (unless spinal trauma is suspected). When he is in dorsal recumbency, check the eyes for nystagmus or strabismus.

- Roll him into lateral recumbency on the opposite side and check the eyes for nystagmus or strabismus.

- Repeat reflex testing on the opposite side, as described.

OTHER REFLEXES

Panniculus

- Test at the cranial edge of the wings of the ilium, progressing craniad until you elicit a response.

Anal Tone

- Check anal tone when taking the rectal temperature, by touching the mucocutaneous junction with the tip of a hemostat or by digital rectal examination.

Flexor Reflex

- When the patient is in lateral recumbency, apply an adverse stimulus to each foot in turn. Weak or absent withdrawal signifies dysfunction of the local motor or sensory components of the reflex.

Crossed Extensor Reflex

- The presence of a crossed extensor reflex in a recumbent animal signifies a lesion ipsilateral to the limb that extends.

BACK OR NECK PAIN

- Check for neck pain by testing range of motion of the neck.

- Check for back pain by palpating the thoracic, lumbar, and sacral spine. Other manipulations may be needed to elicit pain in stoic animals.

Summary of Clinical Signs Resulting From Lesions at Various Sites in the Nervous System

Lesion Location
- Cerebrum
- Thalamus

Clinical Signs
- Changes in behavior and mentation
- Seizures
- Normal gait on a level surface with ataxia and paresis on slopes, stairs
- Contralateral proprioceptive and postural reaction deficits
- Myotactic reflexes normal to increased in contralateral limbs
- Ipsiversive circling
- Ipsiversive head turn (occasional)
- Small pupils, responsive to light (occasional)

Lesion Location
- Limbic system (cerebral, thalamic, hypothalamic, and midbrain centers)

Clinical Signs
- Increased or decreased aggression
- Altered sexual behavior
- Changes in appetite and thirst
- Seizures (often bizarre)

Lesion Location
- Midbrain

Clinical Signs
- Moderate to severely decreased mentation
- Decerebrate posture
- Small pupils indicate mild and/or early lesions
- Dilated pupils with loss of pupillary light reflex and oculo-cephalic reflex indicate severe lesions
- Compulsive circling
- Contralateral hemiparesis to paralysis, ataxia, proprioceptive and postural reaction deficits
- Myotactic reflexes normal to increased in contralateral limbs
- Head tilt away from lesion (rare)

Lesion Location
- Medulla oblongata

Clinical Signs
- Deficits in any of the cranial nerves V-XII
- Head tilt and spontaneous nystagmus
- Decreased mentation (sometimes)
- Ipsilateral hemiparesis to paralysis, ataxia, proprioceptive and postural reaction deficits
- Myotactic reflexes normal to increased in ipsilateral limbs

Lesion Location
- Cerebellum

Clinical Signs
- Intention tremor
- Ataxia in ipsilateral limbs
- Hypermetria
- Decreased to absent menace reflex
- Increased myotactic reflexes in ipsilateral limbs

Lesion Location
- Cranial nerves (peripheral)

Clinical Signs
- A wide range of signs of dysfunction on the ipsilateral side of the head

Lesion Location
- Spinal cord C_1-C_5

Clinical Signs
- Ipsilateral ataxia and paresis to paralysis in fore- and hind limbs with normal to increased reflexes
- Possible urinary incontinence with upper-motor-neuron-type bladder dysfunction

Lesion Location
- Spinal cord C_6-T_2

Clinical Signs
- Ipsilateral ataxia and paresis to paralysis in fore- and hind limbs with decreased reflexes in the forelimbs and normal to increased reflexes in the hind limbs
- +/- ipsilateral Horner's syndrome (preganglionic)
- +/- ipsilateral loss of the panniculus reflex
- +/- urinary incontinence with upper-motor-neuron-type bladder dysfunction

Lesion Location
- Spinal cord T_3-L_3

Clinical Signs
- Ipsilateral ataxia and paresis to paralysis in hind limbs with normal to increased reflexes
- Possible urinary incontinence with upper-motor-neuron-type bladder dysfunction

Lesion Location
- Spinal cord L_4-S_2

Clinical Signs
- Ipsilateral ataxia and paresis to paralysis in hind limbs with decreased reflexes
- +/- urinary incontinence with lower-motor-neuron-type bladder dysfunction

Lesion Location
- Spinal cord S_1-S_3
- Cauda equina

Clinical Signs
- Flaccid paresis to paralysis of the tail
- Urinary incontinence with lower-motor-neuron-type bladder dysfunction
- Flaccid paresis to paralysis of the anus with fecal incontinence

Lesion Location
- Peripheral somatic nerves

Clinical Signs
- Paresis to paralysis of one limb (focal lesions) or several limbs (diffuse disease)
- Rapid muscle atrophy
- Loss of sensation in limbs
- Paresthesias (occasional)

Lesion Location
- Neuromuscular junction
- Muscles

Clinical Signs
- Weakness
- Exercise intolerance
- Muscle atrophy (less common)

Further Reading

Braund KG. *Clinical Syndromes in Veterinary Neurology.* 2nd ed. Mosby-Year Book Inc., St, Louis, MO, 1994.

Chrisman CL. *Problems in Small Animal Neurology.* 2nd ed. Lea & Febiger, Philadelphia, PA, 1991.

De Lahunta A. Veterinary *Neuroanatomy and Clinical Neurology.* 2nd ed. W.B. Saunders Co., Philadelphia, PA, 1983.

Jenkins TW. *Functional Mammalian Neuroanatomy.* 2nd ed. Lea & Febiger, Philadelphia, PA, 1978.

King AS. *Physiological and Clinical Anatomy of the Domestic Mammals.* Oxford Science Publications, Oxford, United Kingdom, 1987.

Oliver JE, Lorenz MD, Kornegay JN. *Handbook of Veterinary Neurology.* W.B. Saunders Co., Philadelphia, PA, 1997.

Oliver JE, Hoerlein BF, Mayhew IG. *Veterinary Neurology.* W.B. Saunders Co., Philadelphia, PA, 1987.

Index